# Gout Cookbook

## Charles Thompson

# Copyright© 2020by Charles Thompson

# Contents

# Gout Cookbook

## Introduction

Well known since ancient times and described by Hippocrates, Celsus, and Galen, gout today affects about 0.3% of the European and North American population. Once considered the prerogative of the wealthiest social classes, it is a disease with a strong genetic component, linked only minimally to lifestyle. Gout is an almost exclusive prerogative of the male sex and begins, on average, between the ages of 30 and 50. A blood test or taking a sample of fluid from the joint swelling can help confirm the diagnosis. A lifestyle change, along with adequate therapy, can keep the symptoms under control. The first attacks generally improve in a few days, but if neglected, the condition becomes the cause of more frequent and painful episodes over the years. The good news is that through the use of specific drugs and an improvement in lifestyle, it is possible to effectively prevent attacks, thus reducing discomfort and frustration in affected patients.

# Chapter 1: What is gout?

Gout is an inflammatory disease that affects the joints and is caused by high uric acid levels that accumulate first in the blood (hyperuricemia) and later in the joints. Generally, gout affects one joint at a time, although in some cases, it can affect more than one at the same time. The most affected joint (75% of cases) is the metatarsophalangeal one of the big toe, but uric acid can also accumulate in other joints and tissues.

## Causes

The cause of gout is the excessive presence of uric acid in the circulation, which generally accumulates for

- dietary causes,
- as a side effect of some medications,
- reduced ability to be disposed of by the kidneys.

To understand how this process occurs, however, it is necessary to take a step back and explain the role of uric acid in our body. Uric acid is a molecule formed from purines, a class of compounds usually present in every human cell and contained in many foods for daily consumption. When the amount of purines becomes excessive, the body can dispose of it by transforming it into uric acid; a waste substance expelled from the body through the urine. This procedure, which we have explained step by step, must be seen as a continuous balance, not as a mechanism that turns on and off as needed; uric acid production is constant, and so is its elimination. It is possible to estimate the amount of uric acid in the body through a blood test (uricaemia) because, in the case of excessively abundant production (hyperuricemia), the disposal systems can go into crisis and thus cause a significant increase in circulating quantities. Beyond a certain threshold, excess uric acid tends to form crystals, just as happens when too much salt is poured into a glass of water. In the beginning, the salt dissolves and disperses in the water (passes into solution) but, by adding a little more, crystals can form, which precipitate to the bottom of the glass.

**Risk factors**

Among the most significant risk factors for gout are:

- familiarity (i.e. close relatives with problems of hyperuricaemia and gout),
- men are slightly more at risk than women,
- excessive consumption of alcohol, because alcohol limits the body's ability to dispose of uric acid, blood levels increase,
- overweight,
- other health problems:
- high pressure,
- hypothyroidism,
- conditions characterized by high cell turnover (psoriasis, anemia)
- prolonged exposure to lead, which tends to raise blood uric acid levels.

It is important to note that so-called modifiable risk factors play a major role in the genesis of the disease; it has in fact been shown that:

- overweight,

- diet
- and alcohol consumption

They are associated with the likelihood of increased levels of uric acids in the blood (and presumably therefore also of gout), even in a direct dose-response relationship (for example, the more severe the overweight, the greater the risk).

Finally, some drugs also increase the risk of hyperuricaemia (high level of uric acid in the blood):

- Diuretic drugs are the class most at risk, because they decrease the body's ability to eliminate uric acid from the blood, favoring its accumulation.
- Salicylates, such as aspirin, can increase uric acid levels in the blood.
- Patients on cyclosporine (immunosuppressant) therapy have a high risk of developing gout.

Under the microscope, the uric acid crystals are pointed and resemble tiny needles. In some subjects, the uric acid crystals are deposited in the joints, while in others, they accumulate under the skin, forming a mass that in some cases can also be felt from the outside and which takes the name of the tophus. Some patients may eventually experience precipitation of urate in the urine, forming painful kidney stones. The immune system, which protects the body from disease, senses the abnormal presence of crystals in the joints and begins to attack them, resulting in the appearance of inflammatory symptoms typical of gout.

# What does gout look like

**Gout is characterized by four stages:**

- Asymptomatic hyperuricemia: High uric acid levels are present in the blood, but there are no symptoms. This phase precedes the first gout attack
- Acute gout attack: Typically occurs following an event that resulted in a spike in uric acid levels. Consequently, once the maximum threshold is exceeded, uric acid crystals are deposited in the joints and give rise to the characteristic symptoms; these usually appear at night, intensify over the next 8-12 hours and then fade over the course of the days until they disappear in just over a week.
- Interval / interaccessual gout: it is the asymptomatic period between one gout attack and the next
- Chronic gout develops when uric acid levels remain elevated for a number of years. This phase is reached in about ten years and is characterized by increasingly severe and frequent attacks that can cause permanent kidney and joint damage.

In most people, the first attack of gout affects the joint of the big toe (podagra), however the joints that may be affected by the inflammatory process are:

- Wrists
- Elbows Instep
- Heels
- Ankles
- Knees

- Fingers

## Symptoms of gout

Initially, gout attacks occur at night or early in the morning, when venous stasis is more marked. They infrequently occur, evolve rather rapidly, and symptoms can persist, if left untreated, for up to one or more weeks.

The most common symptoms with which gout occurs are intense pain, redness, swelling, heat, and increased joint sensitivity.

In some cases, fever, tachycardia, general malaise, and the characteristic tophi (gout tofacea), uric acid nodules that can form in the mucosa, cartilage, or bones of the affected joint may also appear.

## Complications of gout

A characteristic complication of gout is tophi, lumps of uric acid that form in the tissues. The tophi usually appear around the elbows, in the fingers and toes, and later also in other locations such as the ear lobes and Achilles' tendons. In general, tophi are painless, but they can become inflamed so much that, if left untreated, they can cause pain and osteoarthritis, and bone deformities. Chronic uricaemia can also give rise to kidney stones which can block the urinary tract causing infections and impaired kidney function. Furthermore, there is a greater risk of cardiovascular problems in people with gout due to the inflammatory state that can involve different parts of the body, including the heart.

**Prevent gout**

The prevention of gout is based on early diagnosis - especially in those who are familiar with hyperuricemia or who have had gout symptoms at least once - and on the correct management of hyperuricemia through a correct lifestyle:

- Respect a balanced diet and avoid / reduce the intake of foods rich in purines
- Drink plenty of water (2 to 4 liters per day) to help the kidneys avoid uric acid buildup and / or expel already formed stones
- Avoid or limit alcohol and sugary drinks
- Avoid drugs that increase uric acid metabolism
- Maintain adequate body weight and be physically active
- Respect drug therapy

# Chapter 2 Diet and Lifestyle

## Premise

The following indications are for informational purposes EXCLUSIVELY. They are not intended to replace the opinion of professionals such as a doctor, nutritionist, or dietician, whose intervention is necessary for the prescription and composition of PERSONALIZED food therapies.

## Diet for gout

The diet for hyperuricaemia is a diet aimed at reducing the levels of uric acid in the blood; any diet for hyperuricaemia has 4 fundamental characteristics:

- Reduces the intake of purines
- Significantly increases your water intake
- Eliminate any source of ethyl alcohol
- Induces or maintains a normal weight and fights obesity.

**GENERAL DIETARY RECOMMENDATIONS**

Avoid foods with a very high purine content (see later chapters).

Avoid prolonged fasts and highly low-calorie diets, especially those based on reducing or eliminating carbohydrates.

Do not exceed in the consumption of animal proteins, taking 2-3 servings of meat (100 g), 1 of cold cuts (50 g), and 3 of fish (about 150 g) per week. The weights indicated are for illustrative purposes. They should always be calculated as part of a personalized nutritional plan prescribed by a specialist but, in the presence of an underweight or acute inflammatory state, they can be increased by up to 50%.

Hydrate yourself sufficiently, drinking at least 1.5 L of water per day.

Limit fats, drinks, and foods that contain added sugar by consuming at least five servings of fruit and vegetables (three vegetables and two of fruit) every day.

Take sufficient quantities of vitamin C, which, according to some studies, has a preventive role against gout (e.g., citrus fruits, kiwis, strawberries, tomatoes, and raw peppers).

**FOOD NOT ALLOWED**

- Alcohol. Its ingestion (especially beer and spirits), in addition to promoting weight gain, also favors the production of uric acid by the body and its precipitation in the joints. It also reduces its elimination by the kidneys.
- Blue fish with a high purine content, such as anchovies or anchovies, sardines and mackerel.
- Animal offal, such as liver, brain.
- Fatty cheeses, such as those with double or triple cream like mascarpone.
- Shellfish and seafood, such as mussels and clams.
- Sausages, and salami.
- Preserved foods.
- Lard, bacon, cooked or fried.

- Kitchen dice.
- Fructose-containing sugary drinks such as cola and fruit juices.

## FOODS ALLOWED WITH MODERATION

The following are the portions of protein foods suitable for the disease which, however, must be taken according to the weekly frequency of balanced nutrition.

- Meat and poultry (portion of maximum 100 g).
- Cold cuts (portion of maximum 50 g).
- Legumes, such as peas, beans, lentils, chickpeas, broad beans, etc. (portion of 50 grams if dry or 150 if fresh).
- Fish with a medium purine content, such as sea bass, carp, grouper, pike, cod, hake, dogfish, sole, turbot, trout (150g portion).
- Nuts like walnuts, almonds and hazelnuts (10-20g serving)
- Some types of vegetables such as asparagus, spinach, cauliflower and mushrooms.

## ALLOWED AND RECOMMENDED FOODS

- Pasta and rice, breadsticks, crackers, rusks, cereals in general. The starch contained in carbohydrates helps the excretion of uric acid.
- Milk and its derivatives, such as yogurt and ricotta.
- Low-fat cheeses such as mozzarella, scamorza, Parmesan.
- Eggs, 2-4 servings per week.
- Seasonal vegetables . It is good to consume at least one portion of vegetables at each meal, raw or cooked, preferring beets, chard, broccoli, artichokes, thistles, carrots, Brussels sprouts, endive, salad, lettuce, tomatoes, turnips, squash.
- Fresh fruit, remembering however to consume it in moderation for its fructose content (fruit sugar). Some fruits are more sugary than others, such as grapes, persimmons, bananas, mandarins, figs, etc., therefore they should be consumed to a limited extent, while fruits with a low purine content such as apricots, oranges, kiwis, apples, melon, pears, should be preferred. peaches, cherries and strawberries.
- Extra virgin olive oil to season dishes, to be used raw, added in moderation and dosed with a teaspoon so as not to exceed in quantities.
- Water, at least 2 liters per day (preferably natural mineral water).

**BEHAVIORAL ADVICE**

In case of overweight or obesity, it is recommended to reduce weight and waistline, i.e., the abdominal circumference, which indicates the amount of fat deposited at the visceral level. Waist circumference values greater than 94 cm in men and 80 cm in women are associated with a "moderate" cardiovascular risk; values greater than 102 cm in men and 88 cm in women are associated with a "high risk." Returning to an average weight allows reducing blood uric acid levels and reducing other cardiovascular risk factors (such as arterial hypertension, hypercholesterolemia, hypertriglyceridemia, insulin resistance).

Make your lifestyle more active: walk to work, cycle or park far away, if you can avoid using the elevator and walk up the stairs, use a trolley to go shopping and make your way to feet, etc.

Practice physical activity at least three times a week (minimum 150 minutes a week, ideally 300 minutes), aerobic, and muscle-strengthening (anaerobic). Constant physical activity has beneficial effects on those suffering from hyperuricemia and is essential for properly eliminating excess fat and losing weight.

**Diet example**

**Gout Diet Example - Day 1**

DRINK AT LEAST 1.0-1.5 liters of water per day

**Breakfast**

Reduced fat milk 200 ml

Rusks 15g

honey 20g,

**Snack**

Strawberries 200

Low-fat yogurt 125g

**Lunch,**

Pasta with tomato sauce

Semolina pasta 70g

Tomato sauce 100g

Parmesan 10g,

Lettuce 100g

Bread 50g

Extra virgin olive oil 10g

**Snack**

Red cherries 200g

Low-fat yogurt 125g

**Dinner**

Fried eggs

Chicken eggs 100g

Fennel 200g

Bread 50g

Extra virgin olive oil 10g

## Gout Diet Example - Day 2

DRINK AT LEAST 1.0-1.5 liters of water per day

**Breakfast**

Reduced fat milk 200ml

Rusks 15g

Jam, generic 20g

**Snack**

½ Apple, with peel 150g

Low-fat yogurt 125g

**Lunch**

Risotto with zucchini

White rice 70g,

Zucchini 100g

Parmesan 10g

Radicchio 100g

Bread 50g

Extra virgin olive oil 10g

**Snack**

½ Apple, with peel 150g, 52.0kcal

Low-fat yogurt 125g, 70.0kcal

**Dinner**

Ricotta 100g

Eggplant 200g

Bread 50g

Extra virgin olive oil 10g

# Gout Diet Example - Day 3

DRINK AT LEAST 1.0-1.5 liters of water per day

**Breakfast**

Reduced fat milk, 200ml

Rusks 15g

Condensed milk, sweetened 20g

**Snack**

½ Orange 200g, 63.0kcal

Low-fat yogurt 125g, 70.0kcal

**Lunch**

Barley salad with eggplant

Pearl barley 70g

Egplants 100g

Parmesan 10g

Rocket 100g

Italian 50g

Extra virgin olive oil 10g

**Snack**

½ Orange 200g

Low-fat yogurt 125g

**Dinner**

Cod in white

Cod fillets 150g

Chard 300g

Italian 50g

Extra virgin olive oil 15g,

**Gout Diet Example - Day 4**

DRINK AT LEAST 1.0-1.5 liters of water per day

**Breakfast**

Reduced fat milk 200ml

Rusks 15g

Honey 20g

Snack

Strawberries 200g

Low-fat yogurt 125g

**Lunch**

Pasta with peppers

Semolina pasta 70g, 249.2kcal

100g yellow peppers,

Parmesan 10g


Lettuce 100g

Bread 50g

Extra virgin olive oil 10g

**Snack**

Sour red cherries 200g

Low-fat yogurt 125g

**Dinner**

Omelette

150g chicken egg whites

Potatoes 200g

Bread 50g

Extra virgin olive oil 10g

**Gout Diet Example - Day 5**

DRINK AT LEAST 1.0-1.5 liters of water per day

**Breakfast**

Reduced fat milk 200ml

Rusks 15g

Jam to taste 20gl

**Snack**

½ Apple, with peel 150g

Low-fat yogurt 125g

**Lunch**

Carrot risotto

White rice 70g

Carrots 100g

Parmesan 10g

Radicchio 100g

Bread 50g

Extra virgin olive oil 10g

**Snack**

½ Apple, with peel 150g

Low-fat yogurt 125g

**Dinner**

Skimmed milk flakes 150g

Eggplant 200g

Bread 50g

Extra virgin olive oil 10g

**Gout Diet Example - Day 6**

DRINK AT LEAST 1.0-1.5 liters of water per day

**Breakfast**

Reduced fat milk 200ml

Rusks 15g

Condensed milk, sweetened 20g

**Snack**

½ Orange 200g

Low-fat yogurt 125g

**Lunch**

Barley salad with zucchini

Pearl barley 70g

Zucchini 100g

Parmesan 10g

Rocket 100g

Bread 50g

Extra virgin olive oil 10g

**Snack**

½ Orange 200g

Low-fat yogurt 125g

**Dinner**

Baked sea bass

Sea bass fillets 150g,

Chicory 300g,

Bread 50g

Extra virgin olive oil 15g,

# Gout Diet Example - Day 7

DRINK AT LEAST 1.0-1.5 liters of water per day

**Breakfast**

Reduced fat milk 200ml,

Rusks 15g

Honey 20g

**Snack**

Strawberries 200g

Low-fat yogurt 125g,

**Lunch**

Pasta with tomato sauce

Semolina pasta 70g

Tomato sauce 100g

Parmesan 10g

Lettuce 100g

Bread 50g

Extra virgin olive oil 10g

**Snack**

Red cherries 200g

Low-fat yogurt 125g

**Dinner**

Turkey breast 150g

Fennel 200g

Bread 50g

Extra virgin olive oil 10g

# Chapter 3: Breakfast

## 1) Pistachio cookies

**Ingredients:**

- 350 g of Manitoba flour

- 100 g of chopped pistachios

- 150 g of corn malt

- 75 ml of corn oil

- 150 ml of soya milk

- 12 g of cream of tartar yeast

- a pinch of cinnamon

- a pinch of salt

Put the dry ingredients in a container: flour, pistachios, baking powder, cinnamon, salt, and stir. In a mug, mix the malt, oil and 100 ml of soy milk. Pour them over the dry ingredients, work with one hand in a circular direction, mixing the dough and slowly incorporate the rest of the soy milk until the mixture is solid, soft and a little sticky. Let it rest for 15 minutes. Take small amounts of the dough and form balls the size of a walnut. Arrange them on the baking tray and bake them in a preheated oven at 190 ° C for 18-20 minutes or until golden.

## 2)   Muffins with bananas and carrots

**Ingredients:**
- **200 g of wholemeal flour**
- **1 banana**
- **1 medium carrot**
- **milk**
- **60 g of honey**
- **50 g of vegetable butter**
- **1 egg**
- **2 teaspoons of lemon juice**
- **2 teaspoons of cream of tartar**
- **1 pinch of salt**

Gather the chopped butter, honey, and five tablespoons of milk in a small saucepan. Heat them over low heat, stirring until they are homogeneous. Let them cool down a bit. Meanwhile, mash the banana with a fork and coarsely grate the carrot. Mix them in a bowl with the flour, cream of tartar, and salt; gradually incorporate the previously prepared mixture and lemon juice. Finally, add the beaten egg. If necessary, dilute with a bit of milk to have a soft dough. Pour it into paper cups and bake at 180 degrees for about 20 minutes. Allow the muffins to cool on a wire rack before enjoying them.

### 3)  Light pancake

**Ingredients:**
- **100 g of egg whites**
- **125 g of Greek yogurt**
- **80 g of wholemeal flour**
- **2 tablespoons of honey**
- **2 tablespoons of skim milk**
- **1 tablespoon of seed oil**
- **1 teaspoon of baking powder for cakes**
- **1/4 teaspoon of baking soda**
- **1/2 vanilla bean**

**TO SERVE**
- **honey**
- **blueberries or other fruit to taste**

To make the light pancakes, first, collect the egg whites in a bowl. Beat them with a hand whisk for 30 seconds. Add the Greek yogurt, vanilla seeds, honey, and oil. Work everything until you get a homogeneous cream. Add the wholemeal flour, sifted with baking powder and baking soda, and mix it by slowly adding the milk. You will need to obtain a smooth and homogeneous batter with a slightly thick but not too thick consistency. Grease a non-stick pan with the seed oil and heat it well, removing the excess oil with kitchen paper. Pour a ladle of batter and let it spread out into a disc. When you notice large bubbles appear on the surface, turn the pancake and continue cooking on the other side. When cooked, transfer to a plate. Proceed in this way until the batter is used up. Serve the light pancakes warm with honey and blueberries.

**4) Dark chocolate, almond and matcha mini-cupcake without baking**

**Ingredients:**
- **200 g of 70% dark chocolate**
- **1 large handful of shelled almonds**
- **matcha tea**
- **a few pinches of Himalayan salt**
- **a few pinches of vanilla powder**

Melt the dark chocolate in a double boiler. As soon as it has liquefied, add the chopped or chopped almonds, 2 teaspoons of matcha tea, salt, vanilla, and mix well. Pour the mixture into small molds for chocolates or into molds for molds in which you have inserted cupcake cases. Let it cool to room temperature or in the refrigerator. When the cakes have completely solidified, decorate them with a sprinkling of matcha tea.

### 5)   Lemon cookies

**Ingredients:**
**•2 cups of wholemeal flour**
**•2 cups of white flour**
**•3/4 cup corn oil**
**•a pinch of salt**
**•the grated peel of 3 organic lemons**

For the dough's excellent result and speed up the times, it is good to use cold, iced water and work the dough as little as possible. Gather the flours, salt, and peel of 3 lemons in a bowl, pour the oil in the center, and enough water to obtain a thick and creamy mixture. The dough should be rolled out immediately and roughly cut into diamond shapes to get many irregular biscuits. Bake in a hot oven at 200 degrees for 10 minutes.

## 6)   Turmeric pumpkin bread

**Ingredients**
- **700 grams of wholemeal flour**
- **350 grams of pumpkin**
- **200 grams of sourdough**
- **half a cup of sunflower oil**
- **1 tablespoon of whole sea salt**
- **1 tablespoon of turmeric**
- **250-300 ml of warm water**

Steam the pumpkin and mash it with a potato masher, collecting the past in a bowl. Add the rest of the ingredients and work the dough vigorously on a pastry board for 15 minutes. Grease a pan with a diameter of 30 cm, arrange the dough by covering it with a cloth, and let it rise in the heat for 2 hours. Meanwhile, preheat the oven to 230 ° C, or 210 ° C if it is ventilated, placing a steel basin filled with water in the lower part. Brush the dough with water and bake the bread. After 30 minutes, lower the temperature by 30 ° C and continue cooking for another 15 minutes. Remove from the oven and allow to cool before enjoying.

## 7)   Pear, chocolate and hazelnut muffins

**Ingredients:**
- **3 cups of kamut flour**
- **2 tablespoons of cream of tartar**
- **half a teaspoon of ground cinnamon**
- **half a cup of toasted hazelnuts**
- **half a cup of dark chocolate**
- **half a cup of sunflower oil**
- **half a cup of wheat malt**
- **1 and a half cups of soy milk**
- **1 large cup of pears cut into small pieces**
- **1 pinch of salt**

Mix the flour, salt, cream of tartar, and cinnamon in a bowl; in another, emulsify the oil with the malt and milk, then pour it into the first, mixing everything without mixing too much. Add the coarsely chopped hazelnuts and chocolate, the peeled and chopped pears. Spread the mixture into muffin cups and bake at 180 degrees for about 30 minutes.

### 8) Orange Plumcake

**Ingredients:**
- 2 eggs at room temperature
- 170 g of granulated sugar
- 160 ml of orange juice
- 80 ml of seed oil
- 210 g of flour 00
- 50 g of potato starch
- 16 g of baking powder for cakes
- 1 pinch of cinnamon
- 2 organic blood oranges

Start preparing the orange plum cake by whipping the eggs with sugar and cinnamon in the planetary mixer or a large bowl until you get a frothy mixture. Add the finely grated zest of 1 orange and mix. Then add the seed oil and the orange juice, filtered through a colander, taking care to incorporate them well. Continue with the sifted flour together with the starch and baking powder. Pour half of the mixture into a 25x11 cm loaf pan. Place 4 or 5 thinly sliced orange halves on top, cover with the remaining mixture, and spread other orange slices in half on the surface. Transfer to a preheated oven at 180 degrees for about 45 minutes. At the end of cooking, do the classic "toothpick test" to make sure that the cake is ready. Remove the orange plum cake from the oven and let it cool completely before turning it out of the mold and serving.

### 9)  Carrot and raisin muffins

**Ingredients:**
- **250 g of carrots**
- **150 g of kamut flour**
- **150 g of corn flour**
- **2 teaspoons of cream of tartar**
- **70 ml of agave juice**
- **100-120 ml of natural apple juice with no added sugar**
- **100 ml of natural vegetable cream with no added sugar**
- **90 ml of organic sunflower oil (or extra virgin olive oil)**
- **half a teaspoon of dried ginger powder**
- **1 pinch of salt**
- **2 handfuls of raisins**

Preheat the oven to 180 degrees. Soak the raisins in water and leave them for about 15 minutes. Peel and grate the carrots in a bowl. In another bowl, combine the Kamut flour, the cornflour, the cream of tartar, the salt, and the ginger. Separately, in yet another container, pour the oil, agave, apple juice, and cream. Beat with a whisk and add the liquid mixture to the flours.

Mix and incorporate the grated carrots and raisins. Mix the dough. Pour the mixture into the muffin molds using a spoon. Bake and cook for 45-50 minutes or until the surface is slightly colored and the inside is dry enough. Remove from the oven, transfer to a wire rack, and cool for about 5 minutes before unmolding.

## 10) Kamut cookies

**Ingredients:**
- 500 g of kamut flour
- 200 g of corn malt
- 100 ml of corn oil
- 200 ml of warm water
- 50 g of grated coconut
- 20 g of baking powder for cakes
- 5 g of salt

Put the dry ingredients in a container: flour, coconut, yeast, salt, and; mix them well. Mix the malt, oil, and warm water, pour it all over the dry ingredients, and work with one hand in a circular direction, mixing the mixture well. Flour the work surface, place the dough on it and continue to knead until you get a homogeneous, soft, and elastic dough (add a little water if necessary). After a few minutes, roll out a sheet of about 1 cm thick sheet with a rolling pin, then form many biscuits with a pastry cutter or knife. Knead the leftover scraps and create other biscuits until the dough is finished. Put the biscuits in the pan and bake them in the preheated oven at 195 ° for about 15 minutes or until they are golden. Let them cool and serve them.

## 11) Brioche with orange carrots and coconut

**Ingredients:**
- 200 g of rice flour
- 150 g of corn flour
- 170 g of maple syrup
- 200 g of carrots already cleaned and cut into chunks
- 100 ml of orange juice
- 100 g of grated coconut
- 70 g lightly toasted sunflower seeds
- 70 ml of sunflower oil
- 70 ml of water

25 g of cream of tartar
- the grated peel of 1 orange
- 1 pinch of salt

Put the carrots in the jar of the food processor with the salt and the grated orange peel. Start grinding, then add the sunflower seeds and continue. Finally, add the oil, orange juice, lo maple syrup and continue until the mixture is well blended. Put the rice flour, cornflour, coconut flour, and yeast in a bowl, mix well with your hands, and then add the mixture in the mixer and the water. Mix until you get a soft dough: lifting a little dough with one hand and letting it go, it must fall slowly. With the pastry bag or with a spoon, fill three-quarters of the molds with the dough and bake in a preheated oven at 200 ° for 25 minutes. As soon as they are baked, let them cool before serving.

## 12) Salty muffin

**Ingredients:**
- 130 g of wholemeal flour
- 120 g of corn flour
- 1 small carrot
- 1 piece of leek (the green part)
- soya milk
- 3 tablespoons of oil
- 1 teaspoon of oregano
- 3 tablespoon of mixed pumpkin, flax and sunflower seeds
- 1 sachet of yeast
- salt

Chop the seeds and put them in a bowl. Combine the two flours, oregano, yeast, and salt. Pour in the oil first, then gradually add enough milk to have a soft mixture (about 1 glass). Complete with the diced carrot and the washed and thinly sliced leek. Pour the mixture into a tall, narrow mold lined with baking paper. Bake at 180 degrees for 35-40 minutes. When cooked, allow the muffin to cool, turn it out of the mold and let it cool. Serve with a thick tomato sauce or with chopped and sautéed leeks and carrots.

## 13) Gluten-free pancakes

**Ingredients:**

- 220 g of soy milk
- 1 tsp apple cider vinegar
- 15 g of seed oil
- 1/4 vanilla bean or 1 teaspoon vanilla extract (optional)
- 80 g of buckwheat flour
- 40 g of rice flour
- 25 g of corn starch or potato starch
- 4 g of baking powder
- 15 g of cane sugar
- a pinch of salt
- oil to oil the pan

**TO SERVE**

- Maple syrup
- raspberries or other fresh fruit to taste

To prepare gluten-free pancakes in a bowl, combine the soy milk, vinegar, seed oil, and vanilla. Stir and let it rest. Separately, sift the flours with the starch and yeast. Add the sugar and a pinch of salt. Mix the flours with a whisk, and then pour the liquid mixture. Stir vigorously until the dough is smooth and without lumps. Heat a non-stick pan over medium-high heat and cover the surface with a few drops of oil. When the pan is hot, pour 2 tablespoons of mixture for each pancake. When bubbles form on the surface, and the edges darken, flip the pancakes and cook the other side. Repeat the process until the dough is used up, ensuring that the pan does not get too hot. If so, remove the pan from the heat for a minute. Serve the gluten-free pancakes hot with 2-3 teaspoons of maple syrup and fresh fruit to taste.

## 14) Bread croutons with soy, figs and chocolate

**Ingredients:**
- **1 slice of bread**
- **soy sauce**
- **1 dried fig**
- **dark chocolate**
- **Maple syrup**

Lightly toast the bread. Then spread it with an amount of soy as you like. Spread the fig cut into small pieces or slices on top. Sprinkle with maple syrup and complete with the chopped dark chocolate. Eat immediately.

### 15) Potato omelette

**Ingredients:**

- **Eggs 6**
- **Potatoes 500 g**
- **Parmesan 100 g**
- **Parsley to taste**
- **Salt up to taste**
- **Black pepper to taste**
- **Olive oil as needed**

First, chop the parsley finely with a knife. Then peel the potatoes and cut them into 1 cm slices. Bring a pot full of water to a boil and then blanch the sliced potatoes for 4-5 minutes. Now pour the eggs into a bowl, add the grated cheese, the chopped parsley and then add salt and pepper. At this point, stir to mix the ingredients. Drain the potatoes that have finished cooking, let them cool, and then add them to the egg mixture. Then move on to cooking: in a pan, heat a drizzle of oil, and once it is hot, pour the mixture. Cover with the lid and cook over medium heat for 15 minutes, turning the pan from time to time. When the surface is a little soft but still moist, turn the omelet over on the lid by overturning the pan with a decisive and rapid movement. Slide the omelet back into the pan to cook the other side as well, cover again with the lid and continue cooking for another 5 minutes. After this time, the omelet will be ready; you can serve it hot or cold.

# Chapter 4: Appetizer, Snack, Side dishes

## 1) Grilled red cabbage with vegetable yogurt, almonds and turmeric

Ingredients:
- 1 medium red cabbage
- 200 g of natural and sugar-free vegetable yogurt
- 1 clove of garlic
- 1 handful of shelled almonds
- 1 teaspoon of turmeric powder
- dried rosemary, to decorate
- sesame oil
- freshly ground black pepper
- whole sea salt

Wash the red cabbage well and dry it. Cut it lengthwise, making slices about 1 cm thick and trying to keep them compact. Arrange them on a baking sheet lined with parchment paper, salt them lightly and place them under the preheated grill. Let them brown slightly, being careful not to burn them. In the meantime, coarsely chop the almonds, otherwise chop or cut into slices. Blend the yogurt with the peeled and sliced clove of garlic and a tablespoon of sesame oil. Finally, distribute the cabbage in the individual serving plates, pouring a little of the yogurt sauce, a thread of sesame oil, and the turmeric powder on each slice. Decorate with rosemary and serve immediately.

## 2)   Breaded broccoli

**Ingredients:**
- **2 stalks of broccoli**
- **bread crumbs**
- **1 teaspoon of thyme**
- **1 large egg**
- **1 clove of garlic**
- **2 tablespoons of oil**
- **salt and chilli**

Turn on the oven at 180 degrees. Remove the outer layer of the broccoli and slice the excellent stems to obtain discs. Finely chop the garlic and mix it with the breadcrumbs. Add the paprika, chili, and thyme. Mix well. Beat the egg in a bowl and salt it lightly. Pass the coins first in the egg and then in the breadcrumbs, coating them evenly. Line a baking sheet with parchment paper and brush it with oil. Distribute the coins and bake for 10-15 minutes, turning them once. Remove the coins from the oven and serve them immediately.

**3)   Carrot puree with green olives**

**Ingredients:**
- **500 g of spinach**
- **50 g of dried apples**
- **50 g of raisins**
- **a little pine nuts**
- **1 clove of garlic**
- **extra virgin olive oil as needed**
- **Salt to taste.**

Soak the apples and raisins for about 20 minutes in warm water. Clean and wash the spinach. Blanch them in lightly salted water for a few minutes. Drain them by squeezing them well, and cut them coarsely. Fry the garlic in a pan greased with oil, add the spinach, and after a while, the raisins and well-squeezed apples, pine nuts, and salt. Let it cook over high heat for a few minutes, season with salt, and serve the spinach hot.

## 4)   Fennel in orange cream

Ingredients:
- 2 medium fennel
- 1 cup of cashews
- 125 ml of orange juice
- 2 teaspoons of dried mint
- 1 pinch of chilli
- 1 tablespoon of oil
- ½ teaspoon of salt
- 1 teaspoon of agave syrup

Wash the fennel, cut them into four parts, and, using a mandolin, slice them finely. Sprinkle it with salt and let it rest. Meanwhile, prepare the cream. Put the cashews in the blender with the orange juice, mint, chili pepper, oil, salt, and agave syrup and mix until the mixture is fluid and without lumps. Drain the fennel water and season with the cream.

## 5)   Tofu and carrot skewers

**Ingredients:**
- **200 g of tofu**
- **4 slightly large carrots**
- **salt**
- **oil**
- **soy sauce**

Sear the tofu and carrots, diced in salted water. Prepare an emulsion made with two tablespoons of oil and one of soy sauce. Brush the cubes with the emulsion, and put them on the skewers alternately. Sprinkle with a pinch of salt. Bake in a scorching oven for ten minutes and enjoy the crispy skewers.

## 6)   Tofu and vegetable roll

**Ingredients:**
- **tofu 250 g**
- **1 carrot**
- **¼ of  cabbage**
- **1 onion**
- **a pinch of cumin seeds (optional)**
- **soy sauce**
- **extra virgin olive oil**
- **salt**

Boil some water where you can, then place a steaming basket on top. Thoroughly peel and wash the vegetables. With the help of a robot, finely chop the onion and apart from the carrot. First, stew the onion in a pan with a pinch of salt and then the carrot, finally adds the savoy cabbage cut into strips. In a covered pot, sauté the vegetables for 5 minutes. With the help of a fork, crush the tofu to combine with the stewed vegetables. Adjust the sauce with soy sauce and a pinch of cumin seeds. Place the dough in a damp cloth. Roll it up like a salami, tying the ends with a string to make it tightly closed and compact. Steam it for 10 minutes. When it is cold, remove it from the towel and serve it sliced, accompanied with a grain of cereal.

### 7)   Avocado bowls

**Ingredients:**
- **200 grams of brown rice**
- **4 tomatoes**
- **4 avocados**
- **the juice of 2 lemons**
- **1 cup of vegan mayonnaise**
- **a small bunch of parsley**
- **Salt to taste**

Boil the rice in a saucepan with 500 ml of cold water. Put the lid on, lower the heat to the boil and cook until the liquid is used (40-50 minutes). Transfer it to a salad bowl and let it cool. Finely chop the parsley after washing and drying it. Wash the tomatoes and cut them into cubes, then add them to the rice. Separately, mix the mayonnaise and half the lemon juice, and almost all the parsley. Add this sauce to the rice, lightly salt, and stir carefully. Peel the avocados and pit them, sprinkling them immediately with the remaining lemon juice. With the help of a teaspoon, hollow out some of the pulp to form small cups. Mix the removed pulp with the contents of the bowl. Distribute the rice in the bowls, decorate with the remaining parsley and serve.

## 8)   Vegetable snacks in tofu cream

**Ingredients:**
- 8 radishes
- 2 stalks of celery
- 1 carrot
- 4 lettuce leaves

**For the tofu cream:**
- 150 g of tofu
- 3 tablespoons of apple cider vinegar
- 1 tablespoon of extra virgin olive oil
- 1 sprig of thyme
- Salt to taste.

Carefully wash the vegetables, letting the excess water drain for a few minutes. Divide the radishes in half, cut the celery stalks into chunks, and the carrots into slices. Lettuce leaves, on the other hand, should be kept whole. Blend the tofu with apple cider vinegar, oil, and salt. Fill a pastry bag with the tofu cream and decorate the vegetables to taste. With lettuce, it is possible to prepare stuffed rolls, stuffing and rolling each leaf, stopping it with a toothpick. Serve the appetizers garnished with some thyme leaves.

### 9)   Puffed rice snack

**Ingredients:**
- **60 grams of puffed rice**
- **50 grams of white almonds**
- **50 grams of hazelnuts**
- **30 grams of sesame**
- **30 grams of raisins**
- **4 tablespoons of rice malt**

Toast the rice in a pan over medium heat for almost 5 minutes, stirring constantly. Transfer it to a bowl. In its place, put the sesame (washed and well drained) and repeat the operation until it becomes swollen. Toast the almonds in the oven for 15 minutes at about 130 °. Do the same with the hazelnuts, and as soon as they have cooled, remove the peel. Coarsely chop the dried fruit, mix it with the rice in the bowl, and add the raisins. Heat the malt in a bain-marie, and when it is fluid, pour it over the ingredients in the bowl, pouring the sesame. Mix well, and with just moistened hands, distribute the mixture into 4 cm diameter cups. Put the sweets in a preheated oven at 180 ° for 10 minutes, making sure they do not burn. Once cooled, they will be crunchy. They keep well in a tin box for up to a week.

## 10) Lemon tofu crepes

**Ingredients:**
- **200 g of tofu**
- **1 lemon**
- **1 medium sized onion**
- **salt and oil to taste**
- **2 tablespoons of spelled flour for each crepe**
- **some fresh mint leaves**
- **water q.s.**

Brown the finely chopped onion and, when golden brown, sauté the crumbled tofu. Leave to flavor before adding a pinch of salt and the lemon juice diluted in half a glass of water. Simmer in a half-covered pot. Once cooked, with the heat off, grate the lemon peel. For the crepes' preparation: dilute the flour and salt with the mint decoction (bring the water to a boil with a few mint leaves, then turn off) until fluid, but the dense and homogeneous mixture is obtained. Then pour half a ladle of batter on a frying pan lightly brushed with oil and boiling. Cook the crepe over high heat for 20 seconds on both sides, and turn over. Then proceed with the rest of the dough. Stuff the crepes and serve them.

### 11) Black and white sesame crackers

**Ingredients:**
- **50 g of black sesame**
- **50 g of white sesame**
- **30 g of wholemeal flour**
- **40 g of water**
- **extra virgin olive oil to taste**
- **Salt to taste.**

Put the black and white sesame in a bowl; add half the flour, a pinch of salt, and mix. Then pour a teaspoon of oil, water, and mix. Place a sheet of parchment paper on the work surface; distribute the mixture. Overlap a second sheet and pass the rolling pin through it, pushing it lengthwise, possibly until you get a layer as high as the thickness of the seeds. Transfer to a plate and bake for 5-6 minutes; then take it out of the oven, gently pull the paper off the surface and engrave the sheet still soft with a wheel to divide it into long and narrow two-tone rectangles. Bake for another 12-15 minutes. Remove and let it cool completely; remove from the base with a spatula and separate the crackers gently with your hands.

## 12) Brussels sprouts with pears and walnuts

**Ingredients**
- **350 g of Brussels sprouts**
- **40 g of leek**
- **1 small pear**
- **60 g of shelled walnuts**
- **2 juniper berries**
- **salt**
- **4 tablespoons of oil**

Clean and wash the vegetables. Remove the most damaged leaves from the sprouts and divide them into four wedges; add them to the finely sliced leek, which you will dry for 5 minutes in a pan with 2 tablespoons of oil, half a glass of water, and the juniper. Cut the pear into cubes and coarsely chop the walnuts; add them to the mixture and continue cooking for another 3 minutes. Before removing from the heat, season with salt, season with the remaining oil, and stir.

### 13) Slices of crispy bread with black cabbage and beans

**Ingredients:**
- **200 grams of dry beans**
- **300 grams of black cabbage**
- **10 slices of wholemeal bread**
- **7-8 cm of kombu seaweed**
- **a few sage leaves**
- **3 cloves of garlic**
- **extra virgin olive oil as needed**
- **Salt and Pepper To Taste**

Soak the beans overnight, remove the soaking water and cook them in plenty of cold water, with the kombu, sage and a clove of garlic, possibly in an earthenware pot, for about two hours or until tender. Low fire. Season with salt and pepper in the last 10 minutes of cooking; remove the kombu, sprinkle the beans with a drizzle of oil and set aside. Meanwhile, peel the black cabbage by removing the fibrous central rib, wash it well and cook the leaves immersed in lightly salted water, until tender (the black cabbage can be more or less tough). Drain, season with oil and a grind of pepper. Place the slices of bread in the oven and brown them on both sides. Rub them immediately with the remaining garlic. Place them on a serving dish and cover with the beans and black cabbage. Serve immediately.

## 14) Quick pizzas

**Ingredients:**
**For the dough**
- **200 g of finely ground millet**
- **200 g of rice flour**
- **3 tablespoons of oil**
- **1 teaspoon of salt**
- **1 tablespoon yeast**
- **1 tablespoon of sesame and flax seeds**

**For the filling:**
- **500 g of clean pumpkin**
- **1 sprig of sage**
- **1 sprig of rosemary**
- **2 tablespoons of oil**

For the mini pizzas: Finely chop the seeds. Combine them with the other ingredients in a large bowl and knead with your hands to get a soft and homogeneous mixture. Let it rest for about 1 hour. For the filling. Cut the pumpkin into cubes, sprinkle with chopped sage and rosemary. Cook it in steam or the oven for 15-20 minutes, let it cool, and season with oil. Blend it until you have a cream, helping you if needed with a little water. Roll out the not too thin dough with a rolling pin and cut out discs with the help of a glass; place them on a baking sheet lined with parchment paper and cover with the cream. Bake at 170 degrees for about 15 minutes.

**15) Quinoa with roasted carrots**

**Ingredients:**

• **250 g of quinoa**

• **4-5 carrots**

• **4 shallots**

• **1/2 tablespoon of cumin**

• **1/2 tablespoon of turmeric**

• **1 handful of toasted pine nuts**

• **1 handful of parsley and very finely chopped celery**

• **extra virgin olive oil**

• **salt and pepper**

Peel the shallots and halve them; cut the carrots in four lengthwise and then into chunks. Put the vegetables in a pan seasoned with oil, cumin, and salt. Bake at 180 degrees for about 30 minutes, turning them now and then until they are well roasted. Meanwhile, wash the quinoa well in cold water, drain it in a tightly meshed colander and rinse again; drain well and dry briefly in a pan with two tablespoons of oil, turmeric, and pepper. Pour in boiling water equal to double the quinoa's volume, add salt, cover, and cook over very low heat for 15-20 minutes until the liquid is completely absorbed.

Shell the quinoa well and mix it with the vegetables, also

collecting their cooking juices, with the pine nuts, celery,

and parsley. Serve immediately.

# Chapter 5: Soups and salad

### 1) Black lentil cream

**Ingredients:**
- **200 g of black lentils**
- **1 onion**
- **1 clove of garlic**
- **1 carrot**
- **1 stick of celery**
- **10 cm of kombu seaweed**
- **bay leaf, rosemary, sage**
- **salt and pepper**
- **chili pepper**
- **2 tablespoons of oil**

**To garnish**
- **1 diced carrot**
- **chopped parsley**

Dice the celery and carrot, slice the onion and garlic. Heat a saucepan, pour in the oil, and immediately sauté the latter for a couple of minutes, stirring constantly. Add the remaining vegetables and a pinch of chili. Continue cooking for a few minutes, then add the washed lentils, a liter of water, the kombu, pepper, and a bunch prepared with bay leaves, rosemary, and sage. Cover and cook gently for 40 minutes. Remove the seaweed and the aromas. Add salt, blend, let it boil again for a couple of minutes, and turn off. Boil a little water, add a pinch of salt and blanch the carrot as a garnish for 3 minutes. Serve the soup decorating it with cubes and parsley. Complete with a drizzle of raw oil.

## 2)   Leek and pineapple salad

**Ingredients:**
- **2 medium leeks (white only)**
- **150 g of clean pineapple**
- **1 head of curly salad**
- **1 heart of celery**
- **1 lemon**
- **3 tablespoons of oil**
- **50 g of cashews**
- **1 sprig of fresh mint**
- **salt and chilli**

Wash the salad and dry it, then place it in a large bowl. Add the celery rinsed under the tap and sliced. Then add the leek, cleaned and cut into slices, the pineapple cut into cubes, chili pepper according to taste, the lemon juice, the oil, and salt. Stir well. Coarsely chop the cashews and distribute them on the salad together with the coarsely chopped mint.

### 3)  Pumpkin and beetroot salad

**Ingredients:**
**•400 grams of pumpkin**
**•4 beets**
**•1 tablespoon of balsamic vinegar**
**•1 tablespoon of black sesame seeds**
**•2 bunches of rocket**
**•200 grams of cottage cheese**
**•extra virgin olive oil to taste**
**•Salt to taste.**
**•pepper as needed.**

Put the whole beets with the peel in a baking dish with
half a glass of water, cover, and bake in the oven at 180 °
for about an hour until they become soft (you may need
more water). Also, bake the pumpkin cut into small
pieces, with oil, salt, and pepper, until tender and golden.
When the beets have cooled sufficiently, peel them and
cut them into wedges. Mix salt, pepper, balsamic vinegar,
and oil. Combine the beets, pumpkin, and rocket in a
salad bowl. Add the sauce and sprinkle with sesame seeds
and crumbled goat cheese or smoked tofu cut into small
cubes.

### 4)   Potato and leek soup

**Ingredients:**
- 2 large potatoes
- 2 large leeks
- 800 ml of water
- 1 shallot
- 3-4 tablespoons of extra virgin olive oil
- 1 teaspoon of powdered vegetable broth
- 1 tablespoon of dried oregano
- a few pinches of whole sea salt
- a few pinches of freshly ground white pepper

**For the pumpkin seed pesto:**
- 3-4 tablespoons of pumpkin seeds
- a handful of fresh parsley
- half a clove of garlic
- a few drops of lemon juice
- a tablespoon of extra virgin olive oil
- a pinch of whole sea salt
- a spoonful of water

Heat the oil over high heat in a thick-bottomed pot and let the chopped shallot dry out. Add the diced potatoes, oregano, pepper, and add salt by cooking for a few minutes, constantly stirring to prevent the potatoes from sticking to the bottom. Pour the water and the broth powder into the pot, mix, cover, lower the heat and cook for another 15-20 minutes. Add the thinly sliced leek and continue to cook without a lid for about another 10 minutes, until tender.

## 5)  Spiced pumpkin cream

**Ingredients:**
- **1.5 kg of pumpkin**
- **1 shallot**
- **vegetable broth or water to taste**
- **1 teaspoon of curry powder**
- **3 cloves**
- **2 slices of fresh ginger**
- **Salt to taste.**
- **extra virgin olive oil as needed**

Finely chop the shallot and set it aside. Prepare the fresh ginger by cutting two rounds from the root, remove the peel, and cut them coarsely. Also, prepare the other spices required by the recipe for use. In the meantime, wash the pumpkin and cut it into medium sized pieces without removing the skin. Put the already prepared vegetable broth on the fire (even just the water is fine) and put it to heat so that it is already hot when we add it to the pumpkin. Put a saucepan with two tablespoons of extra virgin olive oil and half a coffee glass of water on the stove: add the shallot, ginger, cloves, and curry. Sauté gently for a few minutes, stirring often. At this point, add the pumpkin cut into pieces, brown it in a pot for a few seconds, add the salt and mix well. Add the vegetable broth or water until it is covered. Cook over high heat for about 20 minutes, add salt, and turn off. Remove the cloves and proceed with an immersion blender, blending the mixture until a soft and velvety cream is obtained. Serve hot with a drizzle of raw oil, a sprinkling of toasted sesame seeds, and croutons.

### 6)   Pumpkin and walnut rice salad

**Ingredients:**
- **100 g of cooked brown rice**
- **200 g of grated pumpkin**
- **1 apple**
- **10 walnut kernels**
- **1 handful of mustard sprouts**
- **2 tablespoons of oil**
- **1 tablespoon of wine vinegar**
- **pepper**
- **salt**

It is a recipe that lends itself to recycling previously cooked rice or other grains. Season the brown rice with crumbled walnut kernels, apart from washing and peeling an apple and pumpkin. Prepare a diced apple and pumpkin to sauté in a pan in a bit of oil and a salt pinch. Transfer the seasoning to a bowl with the rice and walnuts and season everything with oil, vinegar, and ground pepper. To close, distribute the mustard sprouts evenly.

### 7)   Autumn garden soup

**Ingredients:**
- **1 small leek**
- **2 cloves of minced garlic**
- **2 tablespoons of minced ginger**
- **100 g of celeriac**
- **200 g of carrots**
- **200 g of potatoes**
- **100 g of beetroot**
- **about 1 l of vegetable broth**
- **2 tablespoons of chives**
- **1 teaspoon of oil**
- **salt**

Cut the leek in half lengthwise and then into small pieces; the other diced vegetables. Sauté the leek for a few minutes in the oil with a pinch of salt over low heat; add half of the garlic and ginger, cook for a minute. Put the other vegetables in the pot and let it all flavor; then pour in the broth and a nice pinch of salt, bring to a boil and cook covered, simmering over low heat for about 30 minutes. Before serving, sprinkle with the remaining minced garlic and ginger. Garnish the individual portions of soup with finely chopped chives.

### 8)   Cream of corn

**Ingredients:**
- **450 g of sweet corn**
- **1 small white onion**
- **380 g of potatoes**
- **1 teaspoon of vegetable butter**
- **300 ml of vegetable broth**
- **350 ml of oat milk**
- **1 lime**
- **White pepper**

**To garnish**
- **slices of avocado**
- **parsley leaves**

In a high-sided saucepan, soften the butter and brown the onion and peeled potatoes cut into small cubes for 5 minutes, stirring and making sure they do not burn. Then add the drained corn, the vegetable broth, and the oat milk. Bring slowly to a boil, lightly salt, and cook for 30 minutes. After this time, purée everything with a fine-texture vegetable mill, helping with the cooking liquid. The filter will only have to retain the well-pressed skins, especially those of the corn kernels. Otherwise, the flavor will be lost. Stir in the lime juice and make the cream homogeneous. Serve it in bowls decorated with a thin slice of avocado and a sprinkle of pepper; give the final touch with a leaf of parsley.

### 9)   Cream of zucchini and avocado with coriander

**Ingredients:**
- **800 g of small fresh zucchini**
- **1 shallot**
- **1 ½ avocado**
- **1 lemon**
- **2 tablespoons of oil**
- **extra virgin olive oil**
- **350 ml of vegetable broth**
- **fresh cilantro**
- **2 tablespoons of oil**
- **extra virgin olive oil**
- **pinch salt**

Wash the zucchini, trim them, and cut them into rings. Peel the shallot and chop it. Gather the two ingredients in a saucepan in which you have heated the oil. Let it cook for a few minutes, stirring. Then sprinkle with the vegetable broth, add salt and bring to a boil over low heat. Cook for 20 minutes. Now add tiny fresh coriander leaves, rinsed and chopped. Mix everything with the hand blender until the mixture is smooth and homogeneous. Reduce to a puree, add the peeled and pitted avocado with the lemon juice and salt. Incorporate it into the previously prepared cream, now lukewarm. Serve the soup in bowls and garnish with and other coriander leaves. You can cook even longer if you want a creamier texture. In the meantime, prepare the pumpkin seed pesto by finely chopping the seeds with the parsley and garlic and mixing everything with the lemon juice, oil, salt,

and water, with the help of an immersion mixer. . When it
is time to serve the soup, distribute it in individual bowls
and complete with a drizzle of oil and a desired amount of
pesto.

### 10) Millet with broccoli and cauliflower

**Ingredients:**
- **650 g of cooked millet**
- **1 spring onion**
- **1 carrot**
- **1 head of broccoli**
- **a few florets of cauliflower**
- **1 handful of lightly toasted sunflower seeds**
- **1-2 tablespoons of oil, salt**

Finely cut spring onion and carrots; blanch broccoli and
cauliflower divided into small inflorescences, in lightly
salted boiling water, separately and for a few minutes. In
a large pan, sauté the onion in the oil for a minute, then
add the carrot and sauté until it begins to soften, add salt.
Put the millet in a pan and let the flavors blend, finally
add the remaining vegetables and seeds, mix well and
serve.

**11) Spelled and bean soup**

**Ingredients:**
- **200 g of spelled**
- **150 g of white cannellini beans**
- **1 carrot**
- **1 onion**
- **2 sticks of celery**
- **½ l of vegetable broth**
- **2 tablespoons of oil**
- **1 bay leaf**
- **salt**

Soak the beans for 8 hours. In a terracotta pot, season the chopped onion in a bit of water for a few minutes, then add the carrot and celery cut into small pieces. Add the bay leaves, beans, and rinsed spelled to the herbs. Cover them with the vegetable broth obtained using the granular vegetable cube and cook everything in a covered pot over low heat for about an hour. Serve the spelled with cannellini beans with a drizzle of extra virgin olive oil.

## 12) Onion soup

**Ingredients:**
- **400 g of onions**
- **6 slices of  bread**
- **25 g of flour**
- **4 cl of oil**
- **1 pinch of nutmeg**
- **salt**
- **pepper**

Toast the flour in a steel pan. Finely slice the onions and sauté them gently with 1 tablespoon of oil and water. Dilute the flour in 1 liter of water, add the softened onions, a pinch of salt and pepper and cook over low heat for 30 minutes. Meanwhile in the oven, lightly toast the bread. Pour the soup into a baking dish, add 3 tablespoons of oil and sprinkle with the chopped toast. Bake at 180 degrees for a few minutes using the grill to get a crust. Serve very hot sprinkled with a pinch of nutmeg.

## 13) Cold cream of carrots with lemon

**Ingredients:**
- **600 g of carrots**
- **450 g of red peppers**
- **500 g of ripe tomatoes**
- **4 tablespoons of oil**
- **extra virgin olive oil**
- **1 lemon**
- **1 radish**
- **fresh mint**
- **salt**

Wash the peppers, halve them and peel them; Bake them on a baking sheet covered with parchment paper for about 30 minutes at 160 °, until the skin is covered with bubbles and turns brown. Remove them and put them in a paper bag so that they cool while remaining moist. Clean the carrots and cut them into slices. Pour them into a pot with a liter of water to a boil and cook for at least 10 minutes. Drain and set aside the cooking liquid. Mix the carrots until you get a puree. Add the peeled tomatoes, seeded and cut into chunks, peeled peppers divided into strips, lemon juice, extra virgin olive oil, and salt. Start the mixer again and, if necessary, dilute the mixture with a little of the cooking water from the vegetables to make it smooth. Pour the cream into small bowls and garnish with slices of radish and mint leaves; serve it at room temperature or after having cooled it for a couple of hours in the refrigerator.

## 14) Chickpea salad

**Ingredients:**
- **2 cups of cooked chickpeas**
- **1 carrot**
- **10 of dried tomatoes in oil**
- **1 sprig of mint leaves**
- **1 tuft of parsley leaves**
- **1 handful of basil leaves**
- **juice and peel of ½ lemon**
- **2 tablespoons of oil**
- **salt**

After cooking the chickpeas in a pot with plenty of water, cut the carrots into thin slices, chop the aromatic herbs and cut the dried tomatoes into very thin strips. To prepare the dressing in a bowl, mix the lemon juice, lemon peel, and oil; mix well. Put all the salad ingredients in a bowl and pour the dressing. Mix well and serve.

# 15) Cream of celery

**Ingredients:**
- 700 g of celery
- 1 onion
- 1 leek
- 2 medium potatoes
- 1 liter of vegetable broth
- 1 bay leaf
- 1 teaspoon of thyme
- 2 tablespoons of extra virgin olive oil
- salt

Chop the onion, leek, and celery. Put them in a saucepan and cover them with the broth. Let them soften over low heat for about 10 minutes, stirring often. Add the peeled and diced potatoes and pour the remaining broth along with the thyme and bay leaf. When it boils, lower the heat and cook for 20 minutes. Remove the bay leaf and puree the soup with an immersion blender. Season with salt, season with oil, and serve hot.

# Chapter 6: Single Course

## 1) Vegetable crumble

**Ingredients:**
- **2 small zucchini**
- **2 potatoes**
- **1 leek**
- **1 pepper**
- **stale bread**
- **Origan**
- **2 cloves of garlic**
- **salt and pepper**

Preheat the oven to 250 degrees. Clean and wash the vegetables. Make a lot of cubes (the smaller the pieces, the faster they cook). Gather them in a bowl and season with salt, pepper, and a little oil. Separately, with the help of a robot, crush a few slices of bread, along with garlic and oregano. You have to get some breadcrumbs. Transfer all the vegetables to a baking sheet and cover them with fragrant breadcrumbs. Drizzle with a drizzle of oil and bake for 15 minutes.

## 2)   Baked spaghetti

**Ingredients:**
- **350 g of spaghetti**
- **10 cherry tomatoes**
- **1 small eggplant**
- **1 cloves of garlic**
- **200 g of tomato sauce**
- **20 black olives**
- **4 basil leaves**
- **4 tablespoons of extra virgin olive oil**
- **Salt to taste**
- **1 chilli**

Wash the eggplant, dry it and cut it into cubes. Put it in a pan with the peeled and halved garlic, the chopped chili, two tablespoons of oil, and four of water. Add salt and cook for 5 minutes over high heat, stirring occasionally. Add the tomatoes divided into four and continue cooking for the same amount of time. Complete with the sauce, the sliced olives, and the chopped basil. Boil the spaghetti in salted water for the time indicated on the package. Mix them immediately with the sauce, season with salt, and season with the remaining oil. Prepare 4 large pieces of parchment paper and distribute the spaghetti. Close the packets well and bake them at 180∞ for about 10 minutes. Transfer them to plates and serve.

### 3)   Eggplant pie

**Ingredients:**
- **2 large eggplants**
- **2 cloves of garlic**
- **800 g of large ripe tomatoes**
- **1 bunch of basil**
- **1 lemon**
- **a few pitted green olives**
- **4 tablespoons of extra virgin olive oil**
- **salt and chilli to taste**

Blanch the tomatoes, peel them, and cut them into pieces. Put them in a pan with 2 tablespoons of oil, minced garlic, salt, and chili. Make them thicken. In the end, season them with the remaining oil and parsley. Meanwhile, check the eggplants, wash and dry them. Cut them into slices about a couple of centimeters thick, salt them lightly and brush them with a bit of oil. Cook them on a wire rack until soft, then remove and set aside. To serve, line up a few slices of eggplant on a plate and cover with a little sauce. Overlap the others and cover with the tomato and basil, continuing in this way until all the ingredients are used up.

## 4)    Risotto with radicchio and almond cream

**Ingredients:**
- **350 grams of rice**
- **1 onion**
- **1 leek**
- **200 grams of red radicchio**
- **1 liter of vegetable broth**
- **2 tablespoons of almond cream**
- **50 grams of flaked almonds**
- **salt and oil to taste**

Peel and wash the radicchio, cut it into slices, and set it aside. Heat the vegetable broth and keep it warm. Cut the onion and leek into thin slices and sauté them in a saucepan with oil, salt, and 3-4 tablespoons of broth, cover and turn from time to time. Add the rice, brown it, and pour a broth ladle; cook, stirring constantly, and gradually add the broth. When there are 10 minutes left to cook, add salt and pepper to taste. Now incorporate the radicchio (set aside a little for the decoration) and cook it so that it is just crunchy, diluting the risotto with a bit of broth to keep it creamy. Remove from the heat and stir in the almond cream. Serve, garnish with fresh radicchio and a few flakes of almonds.

### 5) Pumpkin rice

**Ingredients:**
- **1 cup of  rice**
- **1 onion**
- **400 g of clean pumpkin**
- **3 cups of vegetable broth**
- **1 sprig of rosemary**
- **3 tablespoons of oil**

Put the rice in a saucepan with 2 cups of broth. Cover and bring it to a boil, then lower the heat and cook slowly for an hour. Meanwhile, finely chop the onion and transfer it to a pan just covered with broth. Let it soften over medium heat for a few minutes before adding the diced pumpkin and rosemary leaves. Pour in the remaining broth and cook over low heat for 10-15 minutes. Add the pumpkin to the cooked rice and leave to rest for 5 minutes. Season with oil and salt, stir, and serve.

### 6)   Broccoli and sweet potato pie

**Ingredients:**
- **300 g of sweet potatoes**
- **400 g of broccoli**
- **2 cloves of garlic**
- **1 bunch of parsley**
- **1 glass of vegetable broth**
- **3 tablespoons of oil**
- **salt**

Peel and wash the sweet potatoes, then cut them into slices that are not too thick. Peel and clean the broccoli; slice the stems and divide the flowers into florets. Finely chop garlic and parsley. Line a baking sheet with parchment paper and brush it with a tablespoon of oil mixed with water. Make the first layer with the potatoes and a pinch of salt, a second with the broccoli and a little more salt, a third with garlic and parsley. Finish with the potatoes and pour over all the broth. Bake at 190 degrees for about 40 minutes. When cooked, season with the remaining oil and serve.

### 7)   Fennel and bean pie

**Ingredients:**
- **the outer leaves of 8 fennel (including the green part)**
- **400 g of boiled beans**
- **4 slices of stale bread**
- **1 bay leaf**
- **4 sprigs of thyme**
- **4 parsley stalks**
- **2 lemons**
- **1 tablespoon of coriander seeds**
- **3 tablespoons of oil**
- **salt**

Blanch the already washed fennel. Drain and let them cool, then cut them into strips. Put them in a saucepan. Add 500 ml of the cooking water (if this is not enough, lengthen it), oil, lemon juice, salt, coarsely pounded whole pimento and coriander, aromatic herbs. Simmer them for 10-15 minutes until they are soft and the liquid has evaporated. Eliminate the laurel. Blend the beans with the help of a bit of cooking water: you must have a fairly soft mixture. Season it with salt and mix it with the beans. Complete with the bread cut into cubes (it will absorb the liquid). Put the mixture in a mold moistened with water and press it well. Turn it out on a serving plate. Wash and chop the green twigs of the fennel and distribute them on the pie.

### 8) Barley and rice with ginger-scented asparagus

**Ingredients:**
- **220 g of hulled barley**
- **50 g of rice**
- **500 g of asparagus**
- **1 piece of ginger (3 cm)**
- **3 tablespoons of oil**
- **salt**

Wash the barley, drain it and soak it (1 cup of barley - 3 cups of water) for about 8 hours. Wash the rice, drain it and transfer everything to the pot with the barley and its soaking water. Cook in a pot for 45 minutes. Meanwhile, peel the asparagus and thinly slice the stem, leaving the tips whole. Cut half of the ginger root into thin threads and grate the rest to squeeze two juice tablespoons. In a pan, heat the oil and sauté the strands of ginger over high heat until they turn golden, then add the asparagus stems and a pinch of salt. Cook for a couple of minutes, then add the tips as well, continuing to mix. The asparagus must remain crunchy and bright in color. Add the cereals, drizzle with ginger juice, mix and serve immediately.

## 9)  Tart of peppers with tomato

**Ingredients:**
•4 large yellow peppers
•400 g of tomatoes
•3 tablespoons of extra virgin olive oil
•a few basil leaves
•salt


**For the dough:**
•200 g of flour 00
•30 ml of extra virgin olive oil
•30 g of toasted sesame seeds
•8 g of fresh brewer's yeast
•1 pinch of salt
•1 teaspoon of malt
•100 ml of warm water

Start by preparing the dough: dissolve the yeast and malt in the water; let it rest for 5-7 minutes. Incorporate the other ingredients and knead them, forming an elastic and smooth dough into a ball. Let it rest for 1 hour covered. Peel the peppers, wash them, halve them and put them in the oven at 220 ° for 15 minutes; peel them and cut them into strips. Blanch the tomatoes, peel and chop them. In a pan, pour a drizzle of oil and cook the tomatoes, ½ ladle of water, basil, salt, cover, and finish cooking for 15 minutes over low heat. Let it cool down. Roll out the dough into a 30 cm disc. Arrange it on the pan; shape the edge with your thumbs, and distribute the cold filling. Bake at 190 degrees for 25-30 minutes. Serve the tart hot or warm.

## 10) Buckwheat flan and red lentils

**Ingredients:**
- **350 g of buckwheat**
- **700 ml of hot vegetable broth**
- **300 g of red lentils**
- **300 ml of water**
- **2 onions**
- **3 tablespoons of oil**
- **1 teaspoon of thyme**
- **Salt to taste**

**1 chilli**
- **50 g of sunflower seeds**
- **1 tablespoon of soy sauce**

Cook the chopped onions and chili in a pan with a bit of oil for 2 minutes. Add the red lentils, water, thyme, and salt, cover, and bring to a boil. Lower to low and cook until all the water is absorbed. Toast the sunflower seeds for 15 minutes in a preheated oven at 170 °. Immediately transfer them to a bowl with the soy sauce and stir until they have absorbed it. Wash the buckwheat, drain well, and heat it in a saucepan greased with oil; add the broth and bring to a boil. Lower to the minimum, add salt, put the lid on, and cook without stirring for 20 minutes or until the water is absorbed. Finally, add the red lentil mixture, stir, cover and continue cooking for 2 minutes. Transfer to the pan, level, and bake at 200 ° for 25-30 minutes. Remove from the oven, let it cool for a few minutes, turn over on a serving dish and remove the parchment paper. Sprinkle the sunflower seeds and serve immediately.

## 11) Vegetable paella with seitan

**Ingredients:**
- **300 grams of brown rice**
- **100 grams of seitan**
- **10 broccoli (or cauliflower)**
- **3 tablespoons of fresh peas**
- **1 onion**
- **1 carrot**
- **2 liters of cooking water for the vegetables**
- **1 teaspoon of saffron powder**
- **2 tablespoons of extra virgin olive oil**
- **Salt to taste**

Boil the peas and broccoli in a pot full of water and set them aside (do not throw away the water). Heat the oil in a low and wide pan, put the sliced onion and brown it, then add the chopped carrot and, after a couple of minutes, the rice and sauté for 2 or 3 minutes. Add the seitan cut into bite-sized pieces, the water kept aside, and melt the saffron. Taste and add salt. Cook uncovered and over medium heat until all the liquid is absorbed. Check the cooking and, if necessary, add a little more hot liquid. Pour in the broccoli and peas at this point. Mix well and serve

## 12) Spelled with mushrooms and pumpkin

**Ingredients:**
- **250 grams of pearl spelled**
- **700 ml of water**
- **1 onion**
- **20 grams of mushrooms**
- **300 grams of pumpkin**
- **Salt to taste.**
- **extra virgin olive oil to taste**
- **a sprig of chopped parsley**

Soak the mushrooms for 30 minutes in warm water, squeeze and slice them thin; keep the soaking water aside after filtering it. Dice the onion and pumpkin. Peel the pumpkin, and cut them into small pieces. Season the onion in two tablespoons of oil, stirring for a few minutes; when they are wilted, add the pumpkin and simmer for 5 minutes. Then add the mushrooms and spelled, add the water (including the soaking water) and add salt. Cook for 30-40 minutes over low heat and with a lid. When the spelled is ready, add a drizzle of oil and mix. Garnish with plenty of chopped parsley and serve hot.

## 13) Pasta with turnip and pine nuts

**Ingredients:**
- 350 grams of short pasta
- 300 grams of turnip greens
- 1 clove of garlic
- 2 handfuls of raisins
- 2 handfuls of pine nuts (unsalted)
- 5 tablespoons of extra virgin olive oil
- Salt to taste.
- 1 pinch of red pepper

Put the raisins in warm water. Clean the turnip greens by removing the hardest and most fibrous parts of the stems. Cut into small pieces. Bring plenty of salted water to a boil, add the vegetables and when the boil resumes, immerse the pasta as well. Meanwhile, brown the minced garlic clove in oil; add the pine nuts, the drained raisins and the chilli pepper, leave to flavor. Drain the pasta, pour them into the pan and mix. Drizzle each portion with a drizzle of oil.

## 14) Millet with pesto and tomato sauce

**Ingredients:**
**•350 g of millet**
**•150 g of basil pesto**
**•120 g of fresh ripe tomatoes**
**•3 spring onions**
**•salt**

Lightly toast the millet in a saucepan. Then cook it in water for about 20 minutes. Meanwhile, in a bowl, gather the tomatoes cut into small pieces and reduce them to the sauce with an immersion blender. Towards the end of cooking the millet, add the tomato sauce, stir, and heat. Clean and slice the spring onions, and add them to a bowl together with the pesto. Mix well. Add the millet with the sauce, combine it with the pesto and the rest of the ingredients, season with salt and serve immediately.

## 15) Vegetable burger with tofu

**Ingredients:**
- **250 g of steamed carrots**
- **170 g of tofu**
- **170 g of medium-grain couscous**
- **170 ml of vegetable broth**
- **chickpea flour**
- **3 tablespoons of oil**
- **salt**

Heat the broth and pour it over the couscous; salty. Stir and let it swell for 10 minutes, then transfer to a mixer with the chopped carrots and tofu and the oil. Blend and compact the mixture with a bit of chickpea flour. Take it a little at a time with wet hands and form mini-burgers which you will place on a baking sheet lined with baking paper and brushed with the remaining oil. Bake the meatballs at 190 ° for about 20 minutes, turning them once gently. Serve.

# Chapter 7: Fish

### 1)   Salmon pasta with leek cream

**Ingredients:**

- **Spaghetti 5 cereals 320 g**
- **Salmon steaks 170 g**
- **Leeks 250 g**
- **Fennel 180 g**
- **Shallot 1**
- **Water 500 g**
- **Orange peel 1**
- **Orange juice 1**
- **Chives to taste**
- **Salt up to taste**
- **Black pepper to taste**

Start by peeling the shallot, then cut it into coarse pieces. Peel the leek, cut it into slices, wash the fennel, cut the hardest base, and slice it thinly. Squeeze the orange juice, grate the zest, and keep both aside. Heat a drizzle of olive oil in a pan and sauté the fennel for a couple of minutes; they must remain crunchy. In a pan with a high edge, heat a drizzle of oil and add the chopped shallot, add the leek, let it brown for a few moments, and then cover with water. Add salt and cook for 20 minutes over medium heat. Place a pan full of water, salted to taste, which will be used for cooking the pasta on the stove. Meanwhile, take care of the salmon: remove any bones from the slice with kitchen tongs, heat a drizzle of oil in a pan, place the salmon and sear it on both sides until it is golden brown; then pour the orange juice. Cover with the lid and cook over medium heat for 10 minutes. When cooked, the salmon will be well cooked and pink; transfer it to a bowl and fray it with two spoons. At this point, cook the spaghetti al dente in boiling water for about 7 minutes (adjust according to the time indicated on the package). In the meantime, take the leeks that will be cooked, transfer them to a blender glass and blend them until you get a fluid cream; if necessary, add some pasta cooking water. Pour the leek cream into a pan and chop the chives. When the pasta is al dente, drain it directly into the pan with the cream of leeks, flavored with chives, pepper and then serve on plates by adding a handful of fennel sautéed in a pan to each portion with a spoonful of salmon, garnish with grated orange zest and enjoy your pasta with salmon and cream of leeks immediately.

### 2)  Steamed cod with green olives and cherry tomatoes

**Ingredients:**
- Cod (clean) 600 g
- Cherry tomatoes 250 g
- Green olives 200 g
- Untreated lemon zest 1
- Thyme 8 sprigs
- Black pepper in grains 5 g
- White pepper to taste
- Salt up to taste

Cut the body of the cod into pieces and place them on a saucer. Then prepare the steamer for steaming: fill it halfway with water and when it has heated up, add the sprigs of thyme, the untreated lemon zest, and the peppercorns. As soon as the water boils, place the steamer basket on top, and when it is hot, add the cod morsels (if you don't have a steamer, you can use a large pot and an aluminum colander). Pour the previously washed cherry tomatoes and green olives into the basket. Season to taste with salt and white pepper powder. Cover the cod morsels with a lid to facilitate steaming and cook for about 5-6 minutes or until the meat is white and tender. Then turn off the heat and gently remove the basket to serve your cod with cherry tomatoes and green olives to serve hot!

### 3)  Baked salmon

**Ingredients:**

- **Salmon steaks 4 pieces (Deprived of bones)**
- **Potatoes 170 g**
- **Lemon zest 1**
- **Lemon juice 25 g**
- **Dry white wine 25 g**
- **Extra virgin olive oil 50 g**
- **Parsley to chop 1 tbsp**
- **Salt up to taste**
- **Black pepper to taste**

Take the salmon and transfer it to a baking sheet lined with parchment paper. Take a reasonably regular-shaped potato, wash it and cut it into thin slices without peeling it: the slices must be no more than 1 mm thick; otherwise, they will not be cooked enough. Now take care of the emulsion: grate the zest of a lemon in a bowl, add 25 g of lemon juice, oil, white wine, chopped parsley, salt, and pepper and mix well with a fork. Season the salmon with part of the emulsion, then cover them with the slightly overlapping potato discs and sprinkle the potatoes with the remaining emulsion on the pan. Bake in a preheated static oven at 180 ° for about 20 minutes, then activate the grill at 240 ° and continue cooking for another 3-4 minutes, until the potatoes are golden. After the cooking time has elapsed, immediately serve your delicious baked salmon!

### 4)  Crispy salmon

**Ingredients:**
- **Salmon fillet (4 of 250 g each) 1 kg**
- **Bread 100 g**
- **1 sprig parsley**
- **Dill 1 sprig**
- **Thyme 4 sprigs**
- **Rosemary 2 sprigs**
- **Lemon zest 1**
- **Extra virgin olive oil 50 g**
- **White pepper in grains 1 tsp**
- **Salt up to taste**

Start preparing the breading: cut the bread into pieces and put it in a mixer, then add the dill, the peeled thyme, the rosemary needles, and the parsley. Pour in the oil, then add the lemon zest, salt, and white pepper. Blend until you get a coarse consistency. Now take care of the salmon fillets: remove the skin and remove the bones with the help of kitchen tongs, then transfer the fillets to a drip pan lined with parchment paper and cover them with the breading, making it adhere well with your hands. After covering the fillets evenly, cook in a preheated convection oven at 190 ° for about 20 minutes. After the cooking time has elapsed, remove it from the oven, and serve your crispy salmon piping hot!

### 5) Cod fillet with ginger

**Ingredients:**
- Cod fillet 400 g
- Salt up to taste
- Black pepper to taste
- Extra virgin olive oil 50 g
- Lime zest 1
- Lime juice 10 g
- Fresh ginger (pulp) 20 g
- Mint a few leaves

**FOR THE RICE**
- Basmati rice 200 g
- Coconut milk 400 g
- Water 200 g
- Coarse salt 1 tbsp
- Cinnamon sticks 1
- Curry 1 tsp

Grate the lime zest in a bowl and squeeze it into juice and pour 10 g into the same bowl. Peel the ginger and grate it, then collect the pulp with a spoon and place it in the bowl with the lime, pour in the olive oil and stir to mix the sauce. Take the cod fillets and place them on a baking sheet lined with parchment paper, salt them and spread the sauce on the surface. Bake in a preheated static oven at 220 ° for 25 minutes. Meanwhile, prepare the rice: pour the basmati rice into a pan, add the coconut milk, the coarse salt, the curry and a stick of cinnamon. Pour in the water, cover with the lid and bring to a boil, then lower the heat and cook for 15 minutes until the liquids are completely absorbed. When the rice has absorbed the liquids, turn off the heat and remove the cinnamon stick.

Meanwhile, the cod will be cooked, take it out of the oven and serve it accompanied with the spiced basmati rice, garnishing with mint leaves.

### 6)  Cod with yogurt and purple potatoes

**Ingredients;**
- **Cod 400 g**
- **Natural white yogurt 120 g**
- **Purple potatoes 200 g**
- **Extra virgin olive oil 60 g**
- **Salt up to taste**
- **Thyme to taste**
- **4 slices bread**
- **Vegetable butter 40 g**

Take the cod fillets, and boil them in a pot for about 10 minutes, until they are white and tender. Pour the potatoes into cold water and cook for about 15 minutes from boiling. Then drain and peel them. In a blender, pour the cod and purple potatoes, peeled and coarsely cut into pieces, add the extra virgin olive oil, season with salt and start blending everything. Keep running the mixer while adding the white yogurt, then work until you get a smooth and whipped cream. Add the thyme leaves. Transfer the mixture to the fridge for at least 10-15 minutes. Cut 4 slices of bread, then take the butter and spread it on the bread, then arrange them on a dripping pan lined with baking paper and toast the slices in a static oven preheated to 200 ° for about 10 minutes, until they are golden brown. Serve your creamy cod mousse with yogurt and purple potatoes on the toasted bread, and add a few thyme leaves.

### 7) Sea bream with carrots and zucchini ·

**Ingredients:**
- Sea bream 2 pieces ( clean )
- Extra virgin olive oil 30 g
- Carrots 150 g
- Zucchini 150 g
- Thyme to taste

Wash and peel the carrots, then trim the ends and cut them into slices of about 5 mm thick. Wash and trim the zucchini, too, cut them in half lengthwise and then further divide each half; finally, cut them into cubes of about 1 cm thick. Pour the oil into a large non-stick pan and when it is hot, place the sea bream inside, then add the carrots, the zucchini, the spring onion, and the sprigs of thyme, and add salt. Cover the pan with a lid and cook over medium heat for 7 minutes, then turn the sea bream with the help of 2 spatulas, being careful not to break them; cover again with the lid and cook for another 7 minutes. Of course, cooking times may vary depending on the weight of the sea bream you will use. The pan-fried sea bream is ready to be served!

## 8)   Steamed sea bass

**Ingredients:**

- **2 sea bass not very large**
- **8 cherry tomatoes**
- **4 small potatoes**
- **2 untreated lemons**
- **1 ginger root**
- **1 clove of garlic**
- **fresh thyme**
- **fresh parsley**
- **extra virgin olive oil**
- **salt**
- **pepper**

To prepare steamed sea bass, remove the entrails, scale, and remove the gills with scissors. In a small bowl, collect the thyme, a little chopped parsley, the garlic cut into slices, the grated peel of ½ lemon, and a grated fresh ginger. Cover everything with a layer of oil and mix. Salt the inside of the belly of each bass and then sprinkle with oil mixed with the aromas using a brush. Place the sea bass in the basket lined with a sheet of wet parchment paper and squeeze them together with the cherry tomatoes cut in half and cover them with the chopped herbs. Cover the surface of each sea bass with one or two thin slices of lemon. Then fill the base pot with water, arrange the peeled potatoes. Place the basket for bunk cooking. Cover and cook about 20 minutes without ever opening. Take the potatoes and arrange them on the serving dishes together with the cherry tomatoes. Put half a sea bass on each plate, drizzle with a round of oil, pepper, and serve.

### 9) Fillet of croaker in mango sauce

**Ingredients:**

- Fillet of croaker in mango sauce
- 4 fillets of croaker
- 2 mangoes
- 1 carrot
- 1 zucchini
- a handful of confit cherry tomatoes
- 1 teaspoon granulated sugar
- White wine
- extra virgin olive oil
- licorice powder
- salt
- pepper

To prepare the umbrine fillets with mango and licorice sauce, rinse and dry the fish fillets very well. Transfer them to an envelope for vacuum cooking, after sprinkling them with a little salt, and arrange them in an ovenproof dish. Bake in a steam oven at 85 ° for about 10 minutes. In the meantime, peel the mango, cut it into slices, and blend the pulp with a tablespoon of oil, a pinch of salt and ground pepper. Cut the vegetables into slices and cook over low heat in a non-stick pan. Cover and cook for about 5 minutes. After this time, add the sugar and blend with the wine, raising the heat. Continue cooking for another 10 minutes on a low flame. Serve by placing each fillet on a layer of mango sauce. Season with a pinch of ground pepper and complete with glazed vegetables, confit cherry tomatoes, and licorice sprinkling.

## 10) Baked grouper

**Ingredients:**

- **4 grouper fillets of 200 g each**
- **1/2 lemon**
- **1 glass of dry white wine**
- **1 red chilli pepper**
- **10 g of salted capers**
- **extra virgin olive oil**
- **salt**
- **pepper**

Preheat the oven to 180 C. Wash and dry the fillets well, salt, and pepper them in moderation on both sides. Place them in an oil-coated oven dish by placing them side by side. Season with a drizzle of oil, sprinkle with white wine and lemon juice filtered through a strainer. Transfer the dish to the oven and cook the fish for 15 minutes. After this time, remove the container and add the well desalted capers and the crumbled chili pepper to the fish.
Continue cooking for 15 minutes, no more; otherwise, the fish risks becoming fibrous, occasionally wetting the fillets with their sauce. Remove from the oven, transfer the fillets to the serving dishes, drizzle them with the cooking sauce, and immediately serve the grouper in the oven prepared in this way.

## 11) Salmon fillet with quinoa salad

**Ingredients:**

**4 fresh salmon fillets with skin of
150/200 g each
150 g of quinoa
40 g of pecans
1 handful of dried cranberries
200 g of valerian
extra virgin olive oil
raspberry vinegar
salt
pepper**

To prepare the salmon fillet with quinoa salad, wash the quinoa several times, then transfer it to a saucepan. Cover it with plenty of water (about 400 ml) and add a little salt to a boil. Leave to cook for about 15 minutes or at least for the time indicated on the package. Drain well and transfer to a bowl. Let it cool down. Add the chopped walnuts, valerian, dried cranberries, and season with a drizzle of oil and raspberry vinegar. Season with salt and pepper and mix. Cook the salmon in a very hot non-stick pan, just greased with oil. Start on the side of the skin for about 2 minutes, turn and cook for 4 minutes (however, adjust according to the thickness of the fillets). The salmon must be very soft and juicy on the inside. Transfer the fillets to their respective serving dishes. You can complete the dish with one of the sauces written in the following chapters!

# 12) Fish burger

**Ingredients:**

    **Cod fillet already cleaned 600 g**
    **Grated lemon zest 1 tbsp**
    **Thyme 1 tbsp**
    **Parsley to mince 1 tbsp**
    **Salt to taste**
    **Black pepper to taste**

**FOR BREADING**

    **Eggs 2**
    **Almond flour to taste**
    **Breadcrumbs to taste**
    **Salt to taste**
    **Black pepper to taste**

Cut the fillets into chunks, place them in the mixer, and chop the cod until you get a homogeneous mince. Transfer the mixture to a bowl and season with pepper, salt, chopped parsley, thyme, and grated lemon zest, mix well with a fork. Place a sheet of parchment paper on a cutting board and start creating the fish burger. With a spoon, distribute the cod mixture inside an 11 cm diameter pasta dish and press it with the back of the spoon so that the mixture assumes the shape of the pasta dish. Remove the pastry cutter and cut the parchment paper around the burgers; thus, you will be facilitated in lifting them without the risk of flaking them. Preheat the oven to 180 C. Now take care of the breading: beat the eggs with salt and pepper. Begin to bread the fish burgers bypassing them first in the flour then in the eggs and lastly in the breadcrumbs. Place the fish burgers in the oven at 180 ° C for 25-30 minutes. Once cooked, drain the burgers and place them on paper towels to absorb excess oil. Your fish burgers are ready to be brought to the table hot!

### 13) Mediterranean-style salmon fillets

**Ingredients:**
- Salmon 800 g
- Dried oregano 1 sprig
- Extra virgin olive oil 30 g
- Salt up to taste
- 1 clove garlic
- Pitted black olives 70 g
- Pickled capers 5 g

In a large bowl, add the peeled and halved garlic and the chopped dried oregano. Add the oil, salt, and mix. Take the salmon steak, remove the bones with tweezers, remove the skin if present; then cut into 4 fillets of equal thickness. Arrange the salmon fillets on a baking dish, and with a teaspoon, arrange the garlic oil. Season with salt, add the black olives and capers. Bake in a preheated static oven at 180 ° for about 15 minutes (if you want to use the convection oven, bake at 160 ° for about 10 minutes). After this time, take out and serve your still warm Mediterranean salmon fillets!

## 14) Trout fillet with spinach

**Ingredients:**
**Trout fillets 4**
**Spinach 200 g**
**Grated Parmesan 20 g**
**Onion ½**
**Salt, pepper, olive oil to taste**

Preheat the oven to 180 C. Chop the onion and put it in a pan over medium heat with a drizzle of oil. Add the spinach and brown them together with the onion, salt, and pepper. When the spinach has wilted, remove from the pan and mince. Grease the oven pan with olive oil and place the trout fillets. Cover the trout fillets with the spinach and sprinkle with the Parmesan. Bake at 180 degrees for 15 minutes and serve.

## 15) Sole flavored with basil and mint

**Ingredients:**

> **Fillets of sole 4**
> **Chopped fresh basil 2 tbsp**
> **Chopped fresh mint 1 tbsp**
> **Garlic 1 clove**
> **Extra virgin olive oil 50 g**
> **Salt and white pepper**

Wash the fish fillets and dry them well with kitchen paper towels. Put a non-stick pan on the fire that you have previously greased with extra virgin olive oil and cook over medium heat. As soon as the pan is hot, place the sole fillets on top. Add a little salt, freshly ground pepper, and the mince you have prepared with the basil, mint, and garlic. Cook 3 minutes per side or until the inside is completely white. Season them with a drizzle of raw oil and serve hot.

# Chapter 8: Meat

## 1)   Chicken in Green Sauce

**Ingredients:**

- **Chicken breast 600 g**
- **Parsley 20 g**
- **Basil 15 leaves**
- **Capers 20 g**
- **Pitted green olives 20 g**
- **Extra virgin olive oil 3 tbsp**
- **White onions 1**
- **Carrots 1**
- **Laurel 4 leaves**
- **Black pepper in grains 10**
- **1 clove garlic**
- **Salt up to taste**
- **Lemon juice to taste**
- **Green salad (optional) to taste**

Start by peeling an onion and peeling and cutting a carrot in two. Place them in about 1.5 liters of water and add the bay leaves and peppercorns. Add salt and bring to a boil. Lower the heat and put the chicken breasts to a boil; they will have to cook for 10 to 20 minutes depending on the meat's thickness, which must be completely white but still quite tender. In the meantime, dedicate yourself to preparing the sauce. In a blender, chop the olives, capers, basil, garlic, and parsley. Add 3 tablespoons of oil and a splash of lemon juice and mix everything. Season with salt if necessary and if the green sauce is too thick, add a little oil, a little lemon juice, or a little water to taste. Then drain the chicken breasts. Put the salad in a bowl, add the chicken breasts' strips, and toss with the green sauce obtained. Chicken in the green sauce can also be served with boiled potatoes.

## 2) Chicken and green beans rolls

**Ingredients:**
- **Chicken breast (8 slices of 30g) 240g**
- **Fresh green beans 100 g**
- **Raw ham (8 slices) 70 g**
- **Salt up to taste**
- **Extra virgin olive oil 15 g**

**FOR THE YOGURT POTATO SALAD**
- **Potatoes 500 g**
- **White yogurt 100 g**
- **Partially skimmed milk 20 g**
- **Chives 3 strands**
- **Salt up to taste**
- **Black pepper to taste**

Pour the potatoes into a saucepan with plenty of cold water, place it on the stove and let it boil, then cook the potatoes for 20-30 minutes depending on their size, doing a test with a fork. The potatoes will be cooked as soon as they no longer resist, at which point drain them and let them cool a little, then peel them and let them cool. Once the boiled potatoes are completely cooled, cut them into pieces of a couple of centimeters. Collect the cubes in a container and pour the yogurt together with the chives that you can cut with scissors and mix. If you notice that the mixture becomes too thick, dissolve by adding 1-2 tablespoons of milk, season with salt and pepper, mix, and place in the refrigerator, covering with cling film. Meanwhile, tick the green beans, then remove the two ends, rinse them under running water and blanch them in plenty of boiling water for 10-15 minutes. Then drain the green beans and let them cool a little, adding a little cold water to stop cooking, so they will remain a nice green color. Finally, arrange the green beans in a bowl and season with salt. Arrange the slices of chicken breast on a cutting board and salt them only on the surface. Just above the center, place a handful of green beans. Starting from the highest part, roll the chicken slice with the green beans in the middle to roll up the meat on itself and thus obtain a roll; repeat the operation for all the other slices. Insert two toothpicks for each roll; in this way, you will be sure that it does not open during cooking. Pour extra virgin olive oil into a pan and when it is hot, place the rolls, turning them over after a few minutes of cooking over high heat and continue to seal the meat well. Let them cool for a few moments, and do not throw away the cooking oil that will be used later. Remove the wooden skewers from each roll and salt the surface that was not previously salted. Arrange the slices of raw ham on a cutting board and starting from the bottom roll the slice all around the roll so that the ham completely covers the roll and does so for everyone. In a baking dish, pour the rolls' cooking juices and place them in them, letting them cook in a static oven preheated to 180 ° for 15 minutes. As soon as the chicken and green bean rolls are cooked, you can serve them with your yogurt potato salad!

### 3) Turkey steak with fennel and pomegranate

**Ingredients:**
- **Whole turkey breast 800 g**
- **Fennel 400 g**
- **Pomegranate (1 medium) 400 g**
- **Extra virgin olive oil 80 g**
- **Black pepper to taste**
- **Salt up to taste**
- **Dill to taste**
- **Salt to taste**

On a hot plate, pour a drizzle of oil. Place the turkey on it and cook over medium heat on the first side for about 25 minutes. After the first 25 minutes, turn it over and cook for another 25 on the other side. In the meantime, prepare the dressing: take the pomegranate, cut it in half and shell it, collecting the beans in a bowl; keep some aside for the final decoration, pour the others into a mixer, and blend. Then pass the puree obtained through a colander to filter the juice you can put in a tall glass. Add 40 g of oil, salt, and pepper. Blend everything. Wash and trim the fennel to remove the green part. Divide it in half, then slice it finely, then transfer it to a bowl to the season with 30 g of oil, salt, and pepper. Flavor with the chopped dill with your hands. Stir and spread on a serving dish. Take the turkey, cut it to a thickness of about 1 cm for each slice, and distribute it on the bed of fennel. Season with the pomegranate seeds kept aside sprinkle with the pomegranate and oil emulsion; your sliced turkey with fennel and pomegranate is ready to be served.

**4)  Spiced beef and Parmesan salad**

Ingredients:
- **Fillet of beef 250 g**
- **Cucumbers 300 g**
- **Datterini tomatoes 250 g**
- **Parmesan flakes 40 g**
- **Mint to taste**
- **Extra virgin olive oil as needed**
- **Salt up to taste**
- **Black pepper to taste**

**FOR MARINATING**
- **Extra virgin olive oil 60 g**
- **Mint 3 leaves**
- **Thyme 1 sprig**
- **Pink pepper to taste**
- **Black pepper to taste**

First, prepare the meat's marinade: pour the olive oil into a tall, narrow glass, add the mint leaves, thyme, pink pepper, and black pepper and blend with an immersion blender until you get a homogeneous consistency. Clean the beef fillet by removing any parts of fat or connective tissue, then transfer it to a container and pour the emulsion of oil and aromatic herbs inside. Cover with cling film and leave to marinate at room temperature for about 15 minutes. You can turn the meat when 6-7 minutes have passed so that the other side of the meat can also be dipped well in the marinade. In the meantime, wash and then divide the cherry tomatoes into 4 parts, peel the cucumber, and cut it into thin slices with a potato peeler's help. Place the cucumbers in a bowl and add the chopped tomatoes. After the marinating time has elapsed, cook the fillet on a hot plate for about 3-4 minutes per side. Transfer the fillet to a cutting board, let it rest for a few seconds and cut it crosswise into thin slices. Now you can complete the salad: place the slices of meat on top of the cucumbers and tomatoes, add the flakes of Parmesan cheese, season with a drizzle of oil, salt, and pepper, and, finally, garnish with a few leaves of fresh mint!

### 5)   Veal skewers with rocket and scamorza cheese

**Ingredients:**
- **Slices of veal 600 g**
- **Scamorza cheese 200 g**
- **Rocket 50 g**
- **Extra virgin olive oil as needed**
- **Salt up to taste**

First of all, take only the rocket leaves, removing the part of the stem. Wash them under running water and then dab them with a kitchen towel to dry them. Cut the scamorza cheese into thin slices; then beat the veal slices between two sheets of paper and remove any nerves. Spread one of the slices of meat on the cutting board, place the slices of smoked cheese on top and cover with the rocket. Roll the meat lengthwise to form a roll. Insert toothpicks on top of the roll to facilitate cutting and hold the filling in place. Divide the veal roll into 4 parts, gently remove the skewer and insert them inside a skewer stick, piercing the closed part of the meat slice. Make all the others like this until you finish the meat. Heat a pan with a few tablespoons of extra virgin olive oil and place the veal skewers inside. Cook them for 7 minutes, turning them halfway through cooking. Salt and serve your skewers!

## 6)  Turkey burger

**Ingredients:**
- **Hamburger's bread**
- **Ground turkey 600 g**
- **Eggplant 480 g**
- **Copper tomatoes 320 g**
- **Green salad 60 g**
- **Rosemary to taste**
- **Oregano to taste**
- **Thyme to taste**
- **Salt up to taste**
- **Black pepper to taste**
- **Extra virgin olive oil 10 g**

Start with the chopped herbs: rosemary, oregano, and thyme. In a bowl, combine the minced meat and the mince; season with salt and pepper. Knead all the ingredients by hand and let the mixture rest in the refrigerator for 15 minutes. Meanwhile, wash and trim the eggplant by removing the ends. Slice it about half a centimeter thick and arrange it on a well heated and lightly greased plate. After a few minutes of cooking, turn the eggplant discs to cook them on the other side. When cooked, set aside. Leaf through your salad and rinse it thoroughly so that you can remove any soil residues, then transfer the lettuce to a tray with absorbent paper and pat gently to dry. Finally, wash the tomato and after removing the stalk, slice it half a centimeter thick. Take the minced meat from the fridge and place it inside an 11 cm circular pasta bowl that you will have put on a sheet of parchment paper. Then help yourself with the back of a spoon to level the surface to make it smooth and brush each hamburger with a little oil. Arrange the meat medallions on the hot grill, and after 4 minutes of cooking, you can turn them with the help of a spatula to cook them on the other side for the same time. Cut the bread into two parts and then place the two parts on the still-hot grill, letting go for a few minutes. As soon as your sandwiches are hot, move on to the composition: then on the sandwich base lay 3-4 lettuce leaves and 4 discs of tomatoes, 4 slices of eggplant, and finally your meat medallion. Close with the other half of bread, and your turkey burgers are ready to be bitten while still very hot!

## 7)  Chicken with tomatoes and avocado

**Ingredients:**
- **Chicken breast 550 g**
- **Extra virgin olive oil as needed**
- **Salt up to 1**
- **Black pepper 1 tsp**
- **Lime 1**
- **Oregano 1 tsp**

**FOR THE SIDE**
- **Copper tomatoes 500 g**
- **Avocado 200 g**
- **Red onions 100 g**
- **Salt up to 1 tsp**
- **Paprika 1 tsp**
- **Black pepper 1 tsp**

First, cut the chicken breast into slices, beat them with a meat mallet to make them thinner. Transfer the meat to a pan, then season with oil, salt, and pepper. Also, add the lime zest and its juice, finally flavored with oregano. Mix well to flavor. Cover with cling film and set aside until ready for cooking. Now take care of the tomatoes: after having washed and dried them, cut them into wedges, and then cut them into cubes. Peel and chop the red onion. In a bowl, combine the tomatoes and onion. Now divide the avocado in half, cut the pulp vertically, and then horizontally to obtain cubes. Pour the avocado into the bowl. Season with oil, paprika, salt, and pepper. Now go to cooking: heat a grill well, place the chicken breasts, and cook for 5 minutes. Then turn them and continue cooking for another 5 minutes. Once cooked, immediately serve the chicken with the diced tomatoes and avocado.

## 8) Baked meatballs

**Ingredients:**
- **Minced veal 400 g**
- **1 clove garlic**
- **Stale bread 100 g**
- **Parmesan to grate 100 g**
- **Eggs 2**
- **1 sprig parsley**
- **Salt up to taste**
- **Black pepper to taste**
- **Extra virgin olive oil 2 tbsp**

Start by placing the ground beef in a large bowl, then add the finely chopped stale bread crumbs, the grated cheese, and the chopped parsley and garlic. Finally, add the eggs, season with salt and pepper to taste. Mix the mixture well with a wooden spoon so that all the ingredients are well blended. Cover with cling film and let it rest in the refrigerator for at least half an hour. After this time, form lightly crushed meatballs of the size you prefer with your hands. Lightly oil an ovenproof dish and place the meatballs on it. Add a drizzle of oil and bake in a preheated static oven at 180 ° C for about 40 minutes, until the surface is golden brown. Serve the baked meatballs hot!

### 9)   Chicken breast with orange sauce

**Ingredients:**
- **Whole chicken breast 500 g**
- **Orange juice 130 g**
- **00 flour 40 g**
- **Extra virgin olive oil 30 g**
- **Salt up to taste**
- **Black pepper to taste**

**TO ACCOMPANY**
- **Datterini tomatoes 400 g**
- **1 clove garlic**
- **Thyme 2 sprigs**
- **Extra virgin olive oil 25 g**
- **Salt up to taste**
- **Black pepper to taste**

Take the cherry tomatoes, remove them from the twigs and then rinse them, then divide them in half and place them in a colander set inside a bowl so that the excess liquid will drop to the bottom. In a pan, heat the extra virgin olive oil together with a clove of unpeeled garlic, then add the cherry tomatoes and let them sauté for a few minutes. Season with salt and pepper and let it go for a few more minutes, then remove the garlic clove. When the cherry tomatoes are slightly wilted, turn off the heat and add the thyme leaves. In the meantime, divide the orange in half and get the juice; if you want, you can also filter it to eliminate any residual pulp; keep aside. Then take the whole chicken breast, divide it in half, and clean from any fat and cartilage residues. Flour the 2 pieces well and shake them to remove the excess flour. In a pan, heat oil over low heat; as soon as the bottom is hot, arrange the chicken and let both sides brown nicely for a couple of minutes each. Add the orange juice and cook, sprinkling with the juice and turning from time to time. Leave to cook for 10-15 minutes, and halfway through cooking, add salt and pepper. Once ready, arrange the chicken breasts on a cutting board or plate and slice them obliquely, thus obtaining 2 cm thick slices. Garnish with cherry tomatoes, and your chicken breast with orange is ready: still, enjoy it hot!

## 10) Meatballs in sesame crust

**Ingredients:**
- **Minced veal 300 g**
- **Wholemeal bread crumb 65 g**
- **Parmesan (for grating) 50 g**
- **Sesame seeds 50 g**
- **Black sesame seeds 25 g**
- **Eggs 1**
- **Salt up to taste**

Cut the wholemeal bread crumb into cubes, removing the outer crust, and crumble it in a mixer. In a large bowl, pour the veal, mixing them with your hands; add the chopped breadcrumbs, then the grated cheese. Incorporate the egg and season with salt. Mix with your hands until you get a homogeneous mixture. Each and continue like this until you finish the mix available: with our doses, you will have to obtain 38 meatballs. Pour the white sesame seeds into a tray and add them to the black sesame seeds, mixing them carefully. Pass the meatballs over the sesame, making it stick well to the meat. Continue in this way with all the remaining meatballs and, once finished, arrange them side by side on a baking tray lined with baking paper. Bake the meatballs in a preheated static oven at 180 ° for about 25 minutes, seasoning them with a drizzle of oil if necessary. After the required time, take out of the oven and enjoy your sesame-crusted meatballs hot.

## 11) Veal slices with mushrooms

**Ingredients:**
- **Veal (walnut) 400 g**
- **Champignon mushrooms 500 g**
- **Vegetable butter 50 g**
- **00 flour 40 g**
- **Extra virgin olive oil 10 g**
- **Salt up to taste**
- **Thyme to taste**
- **1 sprig chopped rosemary**

Take the veal slices, and with the meat mallet, slice them to make them thinner, flour the veal slices on both sides, and then shake them to remove the excess flour. Now take care of cleaning the mushrooms: with a small knife, begin to remove the earthy part on the stem, scraping it gently until any traces of earth are removed. If the mushroom is clean enough, remove the few earth residues with a brush, do not wash them with water to not spoil them. Slice the mushrooms and set them aside. Now proceed with cooking the meat: In a pan, melt half a dose of butter (25 g), adding the olive oil; once melted, lay the floured veal slices, add salt and brown them for 3 minutes per side or until a crust forms. Once golden brown, let them cool on a plate and take care of the mushrooms: In the same pan in which you cooked the meat, melt the other half of the butter, season with the chopped rosemary, add the sliced mushrooms and sauté over medium heat for two minutes. , then add salt. At this point, add the veal slices browned and kept aside and flavored with the thyme leaves, cook over low heat for a minute, adding a ladle of water if necessary, and serve the veal with the mushrooms very hot!

## 12) Milk chicken breasts

**Ingredients:**
- **Sliced chicken breast 4**
- **Vegetable butter 40 g**
- **Extra virgin olive oil 10 g**
- **00 flour q.s.**
- **Skimmed milk 170 g**
- **Salt up to taste**
- **Thyme 4 sprigs**

Arrange the slices on a cutting board and, using a meat mallet, beat them to obtain thin slices. Arrange the oil and butter in a pan, let it melt gently, and in the meantime, flour the chicken slices. As you move them into the pan, raise the heat slightly and wait about 2 minutes until a nice crust has formed. Then turn the slices, wait a couple of minutes again, pour the milk first, and then the thyme leaves into the pan. Add salt, cover with a lid and let it cook for another 4-5 minutes until the milk has thickened. At this point, you just have to serve your milk-filled chicken breasts still hot!

**13) Turkey chunks with saffron**

**Ingredients:**
- **Turkey breast 600 g**
- **Saffron (one sachet) 0.15 g**
- **Water about 140 g**
- **Extra virgin olive oil 10 g**
- **Potato starch 1 tsp**
- **00 flour q.s.**
- **Salt up to taste**

**FOR THE ASPARAGUS**
- **Asparagus 400 g**
- **Water 100 g**
- **Extra virgin olive oil 10 g**
- **Salt up to taste**

Start by cleaning the asparagus: wash them, dry them, remove the toughest end, cut them diagonally, and keep them aside. Heat the oil in a pan, add the asparagus, add salt and cook over medium heat for 7-8 minutes, adding about 100 g of water to keep the vegetables from drying out. Once they are cooked, keep them aside and take care of the turkey. Cut the turkey breast into strips and then cut them into cubes of about 1.5-2 cm. Heat a little oil in a pan. Meanwhile, flour the diced turkey in a sieve so as to remove the excess flour. Once the oil is hot, add the turkey, let it brown and then wet with about 100 g of water, or just enough to keep the turkey from drying out. Dissolve the saffron in a little warm water and add it to the preparation; add salt, stir and continue cooking; the morsels must cook in total for about 10 minutes; the time may vary according to their size. Make a cream to thicken the preparation: pour a teaspoon of starch into a small bowl, dilute it with a couple of tablespoons of water and mix to obtain a homogeneous mixture. Add the melted starch to the still hot preparation and mix. Your chicken nuggets with saffron are ready; serve them accompanied with a side of asparagus.

### 14) Loin of rabbit mashed carrots

**Ingredients:**
- **12 rabbit loins**
- **5 carrots**
- **Vegetable broth 2 spoon**
- **Oil**
- **Salt**
- **Vegetable butter 1 teaspoon**

Heat three tablespoons of oil, add the diced carrots and two tablespoons of broth, cook, and add salt. Remove and blend until you have a smooth cream. Heat four tablespoons of oil and a knob of butter, place the rabbit loins in it, brown them evenly, salt them at the end. Remove them and cut each loin into two or three pieces. On the bottom of the serving dish, pour the carrot purée and, on top, the rabbit loins. Serve.

## 15) Chunks of chicken in fennel sauce

**Ingredients:**
- **Chicken breasts g 600**
- **Fennel n 3 medium**
- **Garlic cloves 2**
- **Dry oregano 1/2 tsp**
- **Chili powder 1/4 tsp**
- **Chopped onion 4 tbsp**
- **Extra virgin olive oil**
- **Salt and pepper**

In a large skillet, heat the oil and quickly brown the diced chicken over high heat. Brown on all sides, then drain and keep warm. In the same pan, add the chopped onion, garlic, and cook over low heat for a few minutes. Add the cleaned, washed, and thinly sliced fennel. Wet with two water glasses, add the salt, chili pepper, and oregano, cover, and simmer for about 20 minutes or until the water has dried, and the fennel is almost reduced to cream. Bring the chicken back on the heat, stir, and cook for another 5 minutes. Turn off and serve hot.

# Chapter 9: Dessert

## 1)   Raspberry pie

**Ingredients:**
- **2 cups of wholemeal flour**
- **the peel of half a lemon (preferably organic)**
- **1 tablespoon of rice malt**
- **a pinch of salt**
- **1 glass of water**

**For the filling:**
- **300-400 g of raspberries**
- **100 g of fresh ricotta**

Preheat the oven to 180 degrees. In a bowl, prepare the dough for the base of the tart. Mix the grated lemon peel, a spoonful of rice malt or honey, and a pinch of salt with the flour. Dissolve the dough in water (preferably at room temperature) until it forms a firm stick of dough. With the help of a rolling pin, roll out the dough into a low cake pan, lightly greased with oil or covered with baking paper. Then bake in a hot oven (180 degrees) for 15 minutes. When the tart's bottom appears golden brown, remove it from the oven and let it cool for a few minutes. Before serving, spread the fresh ricotta on the base (it is optional to sweeten it with brown sugar or honey) and distribute the washed and delicately dried raspberries with a cloth.

### 2) Coffee Mousse

**Ingredients:**
- **500 ml of rice milk**
- **3 cups of coffee**
- **100 g of cane sugar**
- **100 g of rice flour**

Gather the flour and sugar in a bowl; mix them well. Pour the rice milk with the coffee into a saucepan, slowly add the flour mixture and beat with a whisk until everything is well blended. Put the mixture on low heat and, still stirring, bring it to a boil. Cook it for 3-4 minutes while mixing, then pour it into a bowl and let it cool in a cold bain-marie, stirring occasionally. If lumps form, remove them with an immersion blender. Let the mousse cool in the fridge for 3-4 hours, then serve it in individual glasses or casseroles.

### 3) Cocoa Puffs

**Ingredients:**
- 170 grams of almond flour
- 1 liter of rice milk
- 50 grams of raisins
- finely chopped almonds (or hazelnuts)
- 50 grams of coconut flour
- 2-3 tablespoons of rice malt
- 1 bay leaf
- 1 pinch of sea salt

Bring the rice milk to a boil with the bay leaf. Add the raisins and flour and cook for 15 minutes over low heat, stirring constantly. Turn off the heat, remove the bay leaf, then add the almonds, coconut, and malt. Leave to cool. Shape into balls of 4-5 cm in diameter and roll them in coconut flour. To serve.

**4)   Almond and apricot cake**

**Ingredients:**

• **500g of chopped apricots + other ripe ones for garnish**

• **½ cup of chopped dried apricots**

• **2 tablespoons of agar-agar**

• **2 cups of almond milk**

• **2 tablespoons of almond cream**

• **the grated zest of ½ lemon**

• **1 teaspoon of vanilla**

• **4 tablespoons of corn starch**

• **½ cup of concentrated apple juice**

• **200 g of ladyfingers**

• **Apple juice**

• **salt**

Put the fresh and dried apricots in a pot together with half a cup of water, the agar-agar, and a pinch of salt. Stirring constantly, bring to a boil, and cook for 5-10 minutes. When cooked, add the concentrated juice, then blend. Use a little almond milk to dissolve the corn starch and rest on the heat with a pinch of salt, lemon peel, and vanilla. When it is about to boil, remove it from the stove, add the almond cream and starch, and then let it boil again and turn it off. Blend the apricots, add the cream and adjust the flavor by adding, if necessary, more concentrated apple juice. Cut the ladyfingers at one end and quickly dip them in the apple juice. Arrange them standing along the edge of a mold of about 22 cm and distribute the cutouts on the bottom. Cover with the apricot cream and leave to cool for a few hours. Remove the hinge from the mold and serve the cake decorated with some halved fresh apricots.

## 5)   Strawberry tartlets

**Ingredients:**
**For the shortcrust pastry**
- **250 g of wholemeal flour**
- **50 g of coconut butter**
- **2 tablespoons of rice flour**
- **2 tablespoons of brown sugar**
- **1 teaspoon of ground cinnamon**
- **1 pinch of pink salt**

**For coverage**
- **4 tablespoons of unsweetened apricot jam**
- **2 tablespoons of chopped hazelnuts**
- **½ tablespoon of lemon juice**
- **1 tablespoon of cherry, plum or apricot distillate**
- **400 g of strawberries**
- **1 sprig of mint**

Melt the coconut butter in a double boiler and let it cool. Pour it into the mixer with the other ingredients and sugar. Operate; when large crumbs begin to form, add a few tablespoons of cold water at a time, continuing to knead the dough until it collects into a ball. Wrap it in a cloth and put it in the fridge for 30 minutes. It is using a damp brush, grease 8 molds with a diameter of 10 cm with oil. Obtain from the thinly rolled dough as many discs large enough to cover the molds' walls and the bottom. They will have to adhere everywhere. Prick the bottom with a fork. Cover each tart with a piece of parchment paper and a few dried beans. Bake at 180 degrees for 15 minutes, remove the paper and the

legumes, cook them for another 5 minutes. After another
ten minutes, remove them, and once cold, unmold them.
Heat the jam with the distillate until it is shiny. Turn off
and add the lemon juice. After a few minutes, brush part
of the mixture on the bases. Wash the strawberries, dry
them gently and slice them not too thin. Distribute them
over the dough. Cover with the remaining jam, sprinkle
the surface with the grains, and let it rest in a cool place
for about an hour. Just before serving, garnish the tarts
with mint leaves.

### 6)   Chocolate nut and almond balls

**Ingredients:**
- **200 g of  flour**
- **150 g of walnuts**
- **50 g of pine nuts**
- **50 g of sunflower seeds**
- **200 g of almonds**
- **50 g of flax seeds**
- **100 g of raisins**
- **100 g of dark chocolate in small pieces**
- **400 g of rice malt**
- **1 lemon**
- **1 orange**
- **6 tablespoons of brown sugar**

Soak the raisins in warm water. In the meantime, grate the peel of a lemon and an organic orange and place them in a large bowl. Add the coarsely chopped walnuts and almonds, flax seeds, sunflower seeds, and pine nuts. Stir in the flour, chocolate, and squeezed raisins and mix well with your hands. Then add the malt and continue to mix all the ingredients with energy. Lightly moisten your hands and form medium-sized balls that you will arrange quite far from each other in a baking tray lined with baking paper. Bake for about 10-12 minutes at 180 °. Let cool before serving. Excellent served accompanied by a fragrant compote of apples and spices.

### 7)   Chocolate truffles

**Ingredients:**
- **100 g of dark chocolate**
- **100 g of almonds**
- **50 g of hazelnuts**
- **100 g of dates**
- **50 g of bitter cocoa**

Soak the almonds in a glass jar for at least 3 hours, then add the dates and leave them for another hour. Meanwhile, heat the dark chocolate in a bain-marie. Drain and set aside the almond and date water. We combine the melted chocolate in the jar with the dried fruit and work it all with the hand blender. Incorporate the chopped hazelnuts and place them in the fridge for an hour. If the mixture is too hard, wet it with one or two tablespoons of soaking liquid. We sprinkle the cocoa on a saucer. We take small doses of the mixture and let them fall on the cocoa. We form balls and compact them well, trying to press them as much as possible. Let's put them in small bowls and skewer each ball with a wooden stick.

### 8)   Cake with strawberries and coconut

**Ingredients for the base:**
- **150 g of toasted soy flakes**
- **150 g of oat flakes**
- **50 g of whole cane sugar**
- **60 g of coconut oil**

**Ingredients for the cream:**
- **400 g of silken tofu**
- **250 g of coconut cream**
- **50 g of whole cane sugar**
- **6 g of agar-agar**
- **200 g of strawberries**

First, prepare the cake base, blending the soy and oat flakes with the brown sugar. Transfer everything to a bowl and mix in the coconut oil previously dissolved in a bain-marie. Transfer the mixture obtained to a 26 cm diameter opening pan, leveling it very well, then put it in the refrigerator to harden (at least a couple of hours). Remember, at this point in the recipe, to put the coconut cream in the fridge. When the base is well hardened, it is time for the cream to separate the liquid part of the coconut cream, pour it into a glass, and keep it aside. Whip the fat part with a whisk. Stir in the silky tofu blended with the sugar, mixing with a spatula, and then the agar-agar dissolved in the coconut water kept aside. Blend for a few seconds and spread the cream evenly on the cooled base. Place the cake in the refrigerator for about an hour until the cream has solidified.  At this point, completely cover the cake with the sliced strawberries and put it back again so that it cools down for at least one night.

### 9) Oat flake cake

**Ingredients:**
- **250 g of oat flakes**
- **120 g of type 1 flour**
- **50 g of coconut**
- **180 g of rice malt**
- **75 ml of deodorized sunflower oil**
- **300 g of prunes or dried apricots**
- **1 lemon**
- **salt**

Soak the dried fruit in water for a few hours and then cook it with a pinch of salt until it becomes soft; make a cream of it, undoing it with a spoon, and flavor it with the grated rind of the lemon. Gather the flakes in a large bowl with the flour, salt, and coconut. Add the oil and the malt mixed in another container and mix everything. Grease a pan and distribute half of the dough, pressing it with your hands; sprinkle it with the dried fruit cream and cover carefully with the rest of the dough. Bake at 200 ° for about 50 minutes or until golden brown. To enjoy it better, let the cake cool for a few hours.

# 10) Berries tart

**Ingredients for the tart:**
- 230 g of wholemeal flour
- 40 g of corn malt
- 40 ml of corn oil
- 5 g of fresh brewer's yeast
- the grated rind of 1 lemon
- 60 ml of warm water

**Berries cream:**
- 250 g of corn malt
- 200 g of berries
- 50 g of corn starch
- 250 ml of cold water
- 1 pinch of salt

Start by preparing the berry cream: put the malt, the washed berries, 200 ml of water, and a pinch of salt in a pot. Cook over low heat and mix. Meanwhile, in a bowl, dissolve the corn starch with the remaining water. When the berries reach boiling point, add the water with the dissolved starch and mix with a whisk to prevent lumps from forming. Within a few minutes, the cream thickens: turn off the heat and pour it into a large baking dish to let it cool. Then proceed with the preparation of the dough for the cake. Put all the dry ingredients in a bowl: flour, salt, and lemon peel and mix them. Then form a hole in the center and mix in the corn oil, kneading it with a bit of dough. Also, add the malt and yeast: work carefully, helping yourself with a bit of flour until you get a homogeneous ball.  Continue to knead for a few minutes on a floured work surface: the result must be a smooth

and elastic mixture that you will leave to rest covered
with a cloth for 30 minutes. With a rolling pin, roll out the
pastry forming a 30 cm disk, place it on a baking sheet
lined with baking paper and shape the edge. Pour in the
cold berry cream. Bake in a preheated oven at 200 ° for
40 minutes, until the surface is golden brown.

## 11) Cocoa pudding

**Ingredients:**
- **500 ml of soy milk**
- **4 tablespoons of unsweetened cocoa**
- **3-4 tablespoons of brown sugar**
- **2 tablespoons of corn starch**
- **1 pinch of natural vanilla**
- **chopped hazelnuts to decorate**

Sift the cocoa, starch, and sugar; collect them in a
saucepan together with vanilla. First, add 100 ml of milk,
stirring well to remove all lumps, and then the rest. Over
medium heat, bring to a boil without stopping stirring.
Lower the heat and cook for a couple of minutes more
until the mixture has thickened. Moisten four single-
portion molds and pour the pudding. Let it cool down and
put it in the fridge until completely cooled. Decorate with
the grains and serve.

<h3 align="center">12) Bavarian yogurt with pumpkin</h3>

**Ingredients:**
- **350 ml of natural yogurt**
- **150 g of grated pumpkin**
- **1 tablespoon of honey**
- **1 tablespoon of agar-agar**
- **1 pinch of salt**

Pour the pumpkin into a saucepan with 100 ml of yogurt, salt, and agar-agar; cook for 5 minutes. Remove from heat, let cool and add the remaining yogurt, honey. Stir the mixture well, then pour it into the bowls and let it cool to room temperature or in the refrigerator.

<h3 align="center">13) Quinoa pralines with peach pulp</h3>

**Ingredients:**
- **1 ripe yellow peach**
- **150 g of quinoa**
- **2 tablespoons of brown sugar**
- **7 tablespoons of coconut flour**
- **5 tablespoons of chopped peanuts**

Peel the peach and chop the pulp in the mixer until you get a homogeneous cream that you will put in the fridge. Rinse the quinoa well under running water and cook it in a pot with boiling water for the package's time. When cooked, drain it, put it in a bowl, add the sugar and let it cool completely. Add with the coconut flour and the peach cream until you get a thick and compact mixture that you will work with your hands to make balls with a diameter of about 3-4 centimeters. Roll them in chopped peanuts and put them in the freezer for 20 minutes, then transfer them to the fridge and always serve them cold.

## 14) Strawberry Tofu Mousse

**Ingredients:**
- **200 g of natural tofu**
- **250 g of strawberries**
- **3 tablespoons of 100% gluten-free rice or corn malt**
- **chocolate flakes**
- **some mint leaves**
- **1 tablespoon of lemon juice**
- **water as required**

Prepare a mint infusion by leaving the leaves to infuse for at least ten minutes in hot water. Strain it and use that water to boil the tofu together with three tablespoons of malt for a few minutes. After cooking, let the mixture cool in its water to make it flavor well. Drain and blend the tofu with the clean and chopped strawberries and a tablespoon of lemon juice. Use the infusion water to help you combine the tofu and strawberries well and obtain a soft mousse. Pour the cream into the cups and store it in the refrigerator for an hour. Finally, garnish with fresh mint leaves and chocolate flakes.

## 15) Chocolate pears

**Ingredients:**
- **1 kg of pears**
- **a little cinnamon or vanilla**
- **100 g of bitter chocolate**
- **3 tablespoons of honey**

Peel the pears, halve them and remove the core. Put them in a saucepan with cinnamon or vanilla and cook them slightly covered with water. Then transfer them to a serving dish, keeping the cooking water. Melt 3 tablespoons of honey in a saucepan and pour it over the pears. In its place, put the chopped chocolate with a little cooking water from the pears. Let it melt until smooth, adding more cooking water if necessary. Spread it over the pears and serve.